Fundamentals of Clinical Ophthalmology

Strabismus

Fundamentals of Clinical Ophthalmology series:

Cataract Surgery
Edited by Andrew Coombes and David Gartry

Cornea
Edited by Douglas Coster

Glaucoma
Edited by Roger Hitchins

Neuro-ophthalmology
Edited by James Acheson and Paul Riordan-Eva

Paediatric Ophthalmology
Edited by Anthony Moore

Plastic and Orbital Surgery
Edited by Richard Collin and Geoffrey Rose

Scleritis
Edited by Peter McCluskey

Uveitis
Edited by Susan Lightman and Hamish Towler

Fundamentals of Clinical Ophthalmology

Strabismus

Francis A Billson
*Professor of Ophthalmology, University of Sydney and Save Sight Institute,
Sydney Eye and Children's Hospitals, Sydney, Australia*

Research Assistant
James Wong
Trainee Ophthalmologist, Sydney Eye Hospital, Australia

Series Editor
Susan Lightman
*Department of Clinical Ophthalmology,
Institute of Ophthalmology/Moorfields Eye Hospital,
London, UK*

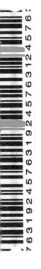

© BMJ Books 2003

BMJ Books is an imprint of the BMJ Publishing Group

First published in 2003
by BMJ Books, BMA House, Tavistock Square,
London WC1H 9JR

www.bmjbooks.com

British Library Cataloguing in Publication Data

A catalogue record for this book is available from the British Library

ISBN 0 7279 1562 2

Typeset by SIVA Math Setters, Chennai, India
Printed and bound in Malaysia by Times Offset

Contents

Preface to the
Fundamentals of Clinical Ophthalmology series

This book is part of a series of ophthalmic monographs, written for ophthalmologists in training and general ophthalmologists wishing to update their knowledge in specialised areas. The emphasis of each is to combine clinical experience with the current knowledge of the underlying disease processes.

Each monograph provides an up to date, very clinical and practical approach to the subject so that the reader can readily use the information in everyday clinical practice. There are excellent illustrations throughout each text in order to make it easier to relate the subject matter to the patient.

The inspiration for the series came from the growth in communication and training opportunities for ophthalmologists all over the world and a desire to provide clinical books that we can all use. This aim is well reflected in the international panels of contributors who have so generously contributed their time and expertise.

Susan Lightman

Preface

This book has been written for the general ophthalmologist, the trainee ophthalmologist, and the eye health professional. It will also be of interest to the paediatrician and family physician.

An increased understanding of the organisation and development of the visual cortex in primates and increased awareness of the interplay between sensory and motor development has resulted in a major shift in the way that clinicians think about infant vision and the eye and child development. The vulnerability of the visual system during development is critical to the understanding of strabismus and amblyopia in childhood and to the presentation of adult strabismus that has its origins in childhood.

There is now an emphasis on development of visual function in early infancy and away from postinfantile development. This has led to concern for development of visual pathways in the cerebral cortex in the central nervous system. Thirty to forty years ago, it was not uncommon for the family doctor to reassure families that a child would grow out of a squint. Now the understanding is that no child is too young to be assessed, managed and treated with the added assurance of safer modern anaesthesia and surgical techniques for infants and children when strabismus surgery is indicated. This goes hand in hand with the understanding that unless treatment is introduced early in the critical periods of development, a good visual outcome will be frustrated. There is now a responsibility for those entrusted with the care of children in the community to become their advocates and to ensure early recognition of abnormality in development, appropriate intervention, and completion of care in their first decade of life.

By contrast, adult onset of strabismus is more often associated with significant underlying pathology in patients with potential for normal binocular vision. Surgical options are similar to those in children except that adults can more often cooperate in surgery and procedures under local anaesthesia. With the implementation of sophisticated treatment, success is often dependent on the presence of a stable substrate of binocular vision and completion within a shorter timeframe.

The opportunity to author this text is welcome because of its challenge to present succinctly the underlying neurophysiologic substrate of binocular vision and strabismus. This perspective provides insights into the vulnerability of the visual system that is the basis for breakdown or failure to develop normal binocular vision. As clinicians, we need to remind ourselves constantly that strabismus is the recognition of a clinical sign, not a diagnosis. Rarely, the disturbed eye movement can be due to a progressive pathological process, for example, neoplasm or inflammation. The primary diagnosis could therefore be a cerebral tumour, threatening not only sight, but also life. The diagnosis of the eye movement disorder would be a secondary diagnosis. The fact that the underlying cause is so frequently static, or a developmental disorder, should not alter the principal of being alert to the possibility of a progressive pathology as the underlying cause. Integration of visual science with observations in clinical practice, and considering the causes and consequences of strabismus through the decades of life should assist us in this.

Francis A Billson

Acknowledgements

I gratefully acknowledge BMJ Books for the invitation to author this text on strabismus and to contribute to this series. The books in this series owe much to the experience of past and present generations of clinicians and scientists who are responsible for creating a discipline within which we are privileged to practise.

James Wong deserves special mention. As my research assistant, James has assisted in the computer generation of this manuscript and as a trainee ophthalmologist, initially in his first year and now into his second year, he has played a further role as devil's advocate, reflecting the initial difficulties those in training have in understanding strabismus. This has led to a simplification of the text and hopefully a clarity that will make this volume useful to the general clinician, registrar in training and specialist in related disciplines.

I also wish to thank Craig Hoyt, Bill Good, and Peter McCluskey. They were generous and patient enough to read the entire manuscript and make incisive comments but any remaining errors are my responsibility alone.

This book reflects the influence of teachers and colleagues. A founding generation for modern strabismus in the last 50 years includes Frank Costenbader, Hermann Burian, David Lyle, Phil Knapp, Marshall Parks, Art Jampolsky, Alan Scott, John Pratt-Johnston, Gunter von Noorden, and Robert Reineke who in turn inspire a present generation. This includes Bert Kushner, Art Rosenbaum, and David Guyton. Those in the discipline of neurology who bring science to the topic of strabismus include David Cogan, John Leigh, and David Zee.

Finally I should like to thank my wife Gail for her support and for patiently enduring my preoccupation with the computer.

Foreword

We should welcome the fine contribution of Professor Francis Billson in *Strabismus* as part of the Fundamentals of Clinical Ophthalmology series. His book reflects his long and thoughtful clinical experience as well as his continued and enthusiastic interest in the basic developmental physiology underlying binocular single vision and the failure of children's eyes to become aligned normally. Professor Billson and his contributing authors have created a relatively small but effective text, terse, direct and simple in style, that crystallizes the essential considerations needed by the clinician to deal with strabismus in all age groups. This book will prove an excellent learning and teaching tool for ophthalmologists that can be read in independent segments or in its entirety. Not only does it provide a survey that gives cohesiveness to the matters of strabismus, but it will refresh, review and consolidate this clinical area for the reader. Hopefully it will encourage ophthalmic surgeons who have shied away from strabismus problems to deal with them more directly with a renewed enthusiasm.

J Raymond Buncic
Professor of Ophthalmology
Chief of Ophthalmology
Hospital for Sick Children
University of Toronto
Canada

Introduction

Medical students have a disturbing way of asking what appear to be simple questions but on reflection are disarmingly penetrating in their focus. Take for example, the medical student who was on our pediatric ophthalmology service recently who dared to ask, "What are the neuroanatomic and neurophysiologic correlates of congenital strabismus?" That we are unable to answer this question in detail is disturbing. However, the breadth of basic science insights into the understanding of the nature of amblyopia and strabismus that have been published in the last few years is impressive.

In this book Professor Francis A Billson, University of Sydney, brings all the recent findings of neuroscience that address the issues of amblyopia and strabismus and places them squarely in the discussion of clinical management of these problems. His ability to blend the science and clinical practice issues relating to amblyopia and strabismus is unique. He details the supranuclear control systems of ocular motor function and places strabismus within the context of a "neurologic" motor disturbance rather than simply an end-organ anomaly. Yet, his discussion is straightforward, concise and ultimately addressed to the clinician. While the reader of this text may not be able to answer the question put forth by our medical student, he or she will have a much more detailed scientific foundation from which to view amblyopia and strabismus. While this text is primarily written for the trainee, even the most experienced strabismus expert will find more than a few insights that will make a careful reading of it worthwhile.

Creig S Hoyt
Jean Kelly Stock
Distinguished Professor
Interim Chair
Department of Ophthalmology, UCSF

Section I
Neurophysiological substrate for binocular vision and strabismus

1 Concepts in strabismus

Normal binocular vision

Normal binocular single vision is the ability of the brain and visual cortex to fuse and integrate the image from each eye into a single perception. It implies bifoveal fusion and a high degree of stereopsis (40 seconds of arc). Normal binocular vision develops after birth from early infancy and is completed with fusion and stereopsis by the age of 8–10 years. Its maturation is associated with a maturation of visual functions in both sensory and motor systems.

Strabismus

- Strabismus is a misalignment of the eyes, such that the visual axes of each eye are not simultaneously directed at the object of regard.
- The misalignment may be present in a particular direction of gaze or in all directions of gaze.
- Strabismus implies an impairment of binocular vision.

The close interrelationship between sensory and motor system development means that strabismus may arise from a disturbance of either sensory or motor development, particularly in the younger patient where the visual functions are more vulnerable.

The near reflex

The concept of the near reflex is important in the maintenance of binocular vision at near and in the effect of refractive error in the development of strabismus. It is also important in the understanding of strabismus and mechanisms of accommodative strabismus. The eye has the capacity to vary its focus from distance to near and this ability (accommodation) is linked in a synkinesis to the power of convergence of the eyes and pupillary constriction in what is known as the "near reflex". The near reflex occurs on visual fixation at near, as in the act of reading. There is evidence that newborn infants can accommodate shortly after birth; as early as 1 month infants are able to intermittently fixate on near targets as determined by retinoscopy.[1] Because of smaller pupils and poorer central vision, newborns have a greater depth of focus than adults and accommodation is not as exact as that seen in later development.

During accommodation the lens of the eye becomes a stronger convex lens in near focus as a consequence of the effect of the sphincter action of the ciliary muscle, relaxation of the supporting zonule and the elasticity of the lens capsule. With greater effort for near focus, there is a greater convergence as binocular reflexes maintain each eye focused on the object of interest.

The importance of the maturity of the near reflex is seen clinically in the Bruckner test which is used for screening amblyopia in strabismus. It is said that in the child, particularly under the age of 4 months, the lack of precision of accommodation prejudices the reliability of the Bruckner test.[2] In the Bruckner test, the eye fixating a direct ophthalmoscope light gives a dim reflex whereas the malaligned eye gives a brighter reflex (see Chapter 6). This test is useful in the child who resents the interference of a cover test. It is important for the clinician to measure strabismus at distance and near with the influence of accommodation controlled. Imbalances between convergence and accommodation do occur and are an important part of the management of strabismus.

Uncorrected hypermetropia in childhood requires increased accommodation. The tendency to overconverge needs good binocular reflexes to sustain control and prevent strabismus. In the infant and young child, the binocular reflexes are immature and the effort of accommodation and increasing power of convergence may result in a breakdown of binocular vision and esotropia. This occurs most commonly at about 18 months to 2 years of age as the child shows increasing interest in the detailed environment. When such a strabismus occurs, it is referred to as an accommodative squint. If glasses correct it completely, it is regarded as fully accommodative. By contrast, intermittent strabismus at distance may be associated with myopia. The myopic patient needs less effort to focus for near. Correcting myopia in these cases increases the accommodative effort needed to see clearly and this strengthens convergence and may, in fact, correct an intermittent divergent squint.

Monofixation syndrome and microstrabismus

Monofixation syndrome (MFS) is a condition where there is suppression of one fovea under binocular viewing. The condition may be primary and without strabismus, although it is more visually associated with a small angle strabismus which is more commonly convergent but may be divergent. MFS may be associated with treatment of strabismus.[3,4] It may be the result of very early surgical intervention for intermittent exotropia, although it is more common after surgical and appropriate spectacle treatment of congenital esotropia.[5]

Microstrabismus may be associated with the absence of bifoveal central binocular vision in the presence of peripheral binocular vision (fusion) and MFS. Documentation of a macular scotoma in a non-fixating eye under binocular conditions is needed to verify the absence of bifoveal fixation. It can also result from anisometropia or macular pathology. It can be the cause of decreased vision in one eye without obvious strabismus.[3,4] A small angle strabismus, usually less than 8 D esotropia, can often be detected under binocular conditions.

Incomitant and concomitant strabismus

Incomitant strabismus is present when the angle of misalignment, measured at a particular test distance, varies. This depends on the direction of gaze and will be greatest in the direction of the impaired muscle movement. Such incomitant strabismus forms a higher percentage of adult onset strabismus than childhood strabismus.

Concomitant strabismus, on the other hand, is more commonly seen in childhood. Simply defined, it means that with accommodation controlled, the angle of misalignment of the strabismus, when examined at a particular test distance, will remain constant regardless of the direction of gaze.

A and V patterns

The terms "concomitant strabismus" and "incomitant strabismus" are descriptive but of limited value in the management of strabismus. Urist (1958) found that almost 80% of patients with horizontal strabismus had vertical strabismus.[6] Concomitant strabismus may become incomitant. For example, in congenital esotropia or exotropia there may be later onset of incomitant strabismus with development of an A or V pattern of movement (Figure 1.1). These patterns represent the changing horizontal

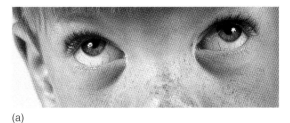
(a)

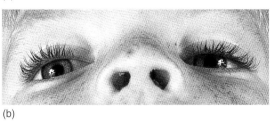
(b)

Figure 1.1 V pattern strabismus demonstrating divergence in upgaze (a) and convergence in downgaze (b). Note the association of hypertelorism in this case

deviation occurring with elevation and depression of the eye. A V pattern of movement, not infrequently seen with congenital esotropia, refers to the fact that convergence is greater in depression of both eyes than in elevation. By contrast an A pattern is the reverse (Figure 1.2). Measurement of an A or V pattern is done at distance fixation. Maintaining distance fixation with the refractive error neutralised, we achieve elevation and depression of the eyes by flexing and extending the neck. If distance fixation is not maintained, simply looking down may induce accommodation and a pseudo-V pattern.

Amblyopia

Amblyopia is poor vision due to interference with normal visual development during a critical period of development. The earlier amblyopia is recognised and treated in the critical period, the greater is the possibility of avoiding poor vision. The importance clinically of the different types of amblyopia lies in timing and ease of reversing the amblyopia. Pattern deprivation amblyopia may occur in the early weeks of life, for example with a dense congenital cataract. The critical period extends for a few months. Strabismic

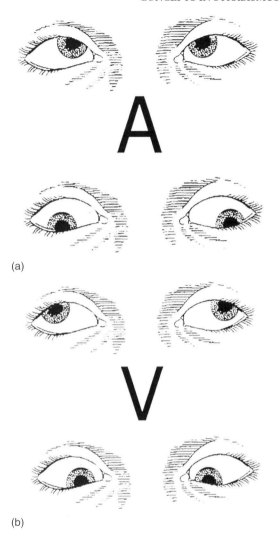
(a)

(b)

Figure 1.2 (a) A pattern strabismus demonstrating convergence in upgaze and divergence in downgaze. (b) V pattern strabismus demonstrating divergence in upgaze and convergence in downgaze

amblyopia may occur some months later after a brief period of ocular alignment. The malaligned eye with an imperfect view of the object of regard is at risk of poor vision because of dominance of the fixing eye. Anisometropia amblyopia is due to difference in refractive error between the two eyes. Its critical period extends until 7–8 years of age. If the eyes are aligned, amblyopia may still develop because of imperfect imaging on the retina of one eye,

5

compared to the image on the retina of the other eye. If in addition to anisometropia the eyes are malaligned, strabismic amblyopia could contribute further to the poor vision.

Strabismic amblyopia is an acquired defect in monocular vision due to malalignment resulting in disturbed binocular vision without an underlying organic cause. The poor vision is a reflection of suppression of visual cortex neuronal function. Strabismus usually precedes amblyopia but poor vision in one eye may be due to structural abnormalities in the retina (for example, retinoblastoma). The damaged retina prevents capture of a clear image, frustrating binocular vision and resulting in squint (secondary strabismus). Poor vision itself results in strabismus because visual development requires clear imaging in each eye for normal development of binocular vision. It follows that "every squinting eye should be regarded as potentially a blind eye", either because the poor vision is due to amblyopia resulting from the strabismic eye, or because underlying pathology is the cause of the poor vision and strabismus is secondary to the inability to establish binocular vision.

Strabismic amblyopia results from malalignment of the visual axes, with one eye preferred for fixation. It is attended by progressive loss of vision in the non-fixing eye. Strabismic amblyopia complicated by anisometropia can occur when difference in refraction determines the fixing eye. Unilateral cataract can be a sensory cause of a strabismus. Early surgical treatment of the cataract and optical treatment with an intraocular lens (pseudophakic correction) can correct the pattern amblyopia. However, the deviation of the eye previously associated with the cataract may be attended by strabismic amblyopia[7] unless the pseudophakic eye is encouraged to take up fixation. Difference in refraction, due to the removal of the lens, may lead to anisometropic amblyopia unless early optical correction with a contact lens or an intraocular lens occurs. Meridional amblyopia is a special case where the astigmatic meridian is suppressed because of the retinal rivalry and dominance of opposing cells in the other eye. Meridional amblyopia can be bilateral when the astigmatism is in a different axis in each eye. A neutral density filter placed in front of an eye with an organic defect reduces visual acuity, in contrast to the filter placed in front of an amblyopic eye, where the vision is not further degraded.

Bilateral form deprivation may occur in the presence of nystagmus. This will depend on features such as interference with foveation time and whether or not there is a null point where fixation can be maintained.

Clinically, critical periods exist for normal visual development. At such times if there is interference with clear imaging in either eye, loss of vision in the affected eye, loss of binocular vision, and strabismus are most likely to occur. These critical periods occur in infancy and early childhood, at an important time when there is great plasticity during the maturation of the visual system and brain. This plasticity extends up to 10–12 years of age, but is greatest in the first 3 months of infancy and under the age of 5, and being less in evidence as the child approaches age 9. The plasticity also implies the changes are reversible. The earlier visual deprivation is treated and reversed, the better the outcome. Uniocular visual deprivation causes more profound change in the visual cortex than simultaneous binocular deprivation.

References

1. Banks M. The development of visual accommodation during infancy. *Child Dev* 1980;**51**:646.
2. Archer SM. Developmental aspect of the Bruckner Test. *Ophthalmology* 1988;**95**:1098.
3. Parks MM. The monofixation syndrome. *Trans Am Ophthalmol Soc* 1969;**67**:609–57.
4. Parks MM. Sensory adaptations in strabismus. In: Nelson LB, Calhoun JH, Harley RD, eds. *Pediatric Ophthalmology*. Philadelphia: WB Saunders, 1991.
5. Good WV, Lyons, CJ, Hoyt CS. Monocular visual outcome in untreated early onset esotropia. *Br J Ophthalmol* 1993;**77**:492–94.
6. Urist MJ. The etiology of the so-called A and V syndromes. *Am J Ophthalmol* 1958;**46**:835–44.
7. Sengpiel F, Blakemore C. The neural basis of suppression and amblyopia in strabismus. *Eye* 1996;**10**:250–8.

2 A simple reflex model of normal binocular vision

Introduction

Understanding normal binocular single vision can be simplified by comparison with a simple spinal reflex with afferent and efferent neurons. The visual pathway represents the sensory arc and the lower motor neurons of the third, fourth and sixth cranial nerves the motor arc of the reflex. The sensory visual centre in the cortex and the motor fusion centre in the brainstem may be likened to the interneurons of the spinal cord participating in the integration of sensory and motor arcs of the reflex. Furthermore, like spinal reflexes, normal binocular vision can be modified by voluntary and involuntary influences (Figure 2.1).

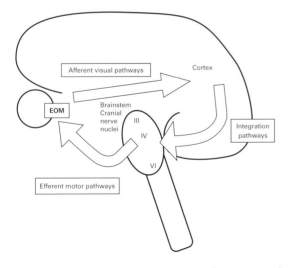

Figure 2.1 A simple reflex concept of sensory and motor integration of binocular vision
EOM = extraocular muscle

Sensory arc (visual pathway)

The sensory visual path comprises the retina, optic nerves, chiasm, optic tracts, lateral geniculate nucleus, optic radiations and visual cortex. Visual information from each hemiretina is paired with that from the corresponding hemiretina of the fellow eye, with the nerve fibres from each nasal hemiretina crossing over in the optic chiasm, an essential requirement for binocular vision. The visual information is processed in an increasingly complex fashion in the association (extrastriate) cortex.

Parallel processing has been revealed by the study of the primate visual system with the information carried in the visual pathway being processed in at least two distinct visual streams: the M (magnocellular) and P (parvocellular). The M pathway subserves motion, direction, coarse stereopsis, speed judgement and smooth pursuit, and appears to play a dominant role in localising and tracking objects. The P stream subserves fine acuity, fine stereopsis, shape and colour, and identifying the precise features of static objects. These roles are relative and overlap in clinical testing to different degrees. These two parallel cellular pathways begin in specialised ganglion cells in the retina and maintain separateness through to the striate and extrastriate cortex (Figure 2.2).

Retina

Visual information passes through the retina to the photoreceptors and is processed in the

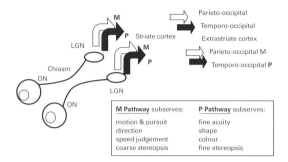

Figure 2.2 Simplified illustration of the sensory visual path demonstrating parallel pathways and increasingly complex visual processing from each eye through optic nerves (ON), lateral geniculate nucleus (LGN), striate and extrastriate cortex

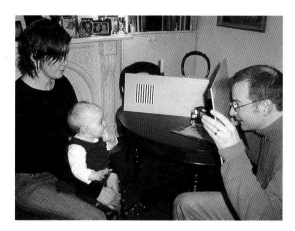

Figure 2.3 A baby's vision is tested using Teller acuity cards, each with varying spatial frequency. Note an example of the card on the table

neural layers of the retina, reaching the magnocellular and parvocellular ganglion cell layers in the inner retina. M and P parallel visual paths project from the M and P ganglion cells in the inner retina and travel in the optic nerve to the lateral geniculate nucleus (LGN).

Lateral geniculate nucleus

The M and P ganglion cells reach separate M and P laminae in the LGN.

Striate cortex (V1)

The M and P paths project from separate LGN laminae to the striate cortex. M neurons project to lamina IVB and P neurons project to laminae IVA, II and III.

Extrastriate cortex

M neurons project to parieto-occipital regions of the extrastriate cortex and P neurons project to temporo-occipital regions. Information then combines into an integrated visual perception, including motion, colour and fine detail.[1]

The clinical significance of this is reflected in the illustration that different visual functions develop at different ages. Studies have shown that at 6 months visual acuity is 6/36 on Teller acuity and continues to improve to 6/6 by age 2 years (Figure 2.3).[2] Similarly, contrast sensitivity for detecting movement and lower spatial frequencies is thought to develop from about 3 months and be mature by 6 months.[3]

Integration components of normal binocular vision

When an individual with normal binocular vision is looking straight ahead at an object in the primary position of gaze, equal visual information is falling on corresponding points of each retina and in particular the macula of each eye. The information is being integrated within the visual centre, the extrastriate cortex, and the information is passed to the motor nuclei of the extraocular muscle via the motor fusion centre in the brainstem.

Sensory integration – extrastriate visual cortex

Hubel and Weisel suggested that the difference between uniocular deprivation and binocular deprivation of vision depended on interaction of information carried in two distinct visual pathways from each eye to the visual cortex.[4] The pathways diverge from the striate cortex so that M-pathway information is conveyed predominantly to more dorsal regions of the extrastriate cortex (parieto-occipital) and P information to more ventral (temporo-occipital) regions.

It is thought that the infantile phase of the critical period during which this information can be realised in the visual cortex begins and ends *earlier* for M-neuron functions (such as large disparity stereopsis and pursuit motion processing) and begins and ends *later* for P-neuron functions (such as fine spatial acuity). The M-neuron functions are present in the early months of life and established by 3–5 months of life. The P-neuron functions begin to appear at about 4 months but do not approach adult level until about 12 months of life. The development of the M and P-neuron functions is mirrored clinically. In the first 3 months of life infants superimpose visual images. At 3 months binocular fusion commences in the form of rivalry aversion.[5,6] Sensitivities to stereoscopic disparity in visual images progressively improve in infants between 3 and 6 months.

Clinical studies using the techniques of preferential looking and electrophysiology have placed the development of stereopsis between the ages of 2 and 6 months.[7,8] This development occurs relatively rapidly and appears to plateau, with less maturation occurring after the age of 6 months. If normal development of binocular vision occurs by age 3–5 months, the more primitive nasally directed pursuit bias is replaced by symmetric nasotemporal pursuit.[9]

Motor integration – motor fusion centres in the brainstem

The development of motor fusion is dependent on the maturation of binocular reflexes in the sensory M stream of the visual cortex; these appear to provide the binocular signals for binocular eye alignment, conjugate eye movement and nasotemporal pursuit.

The exact pathways are not without dispute, but evidence from primate monkey recordings and suggestive evidence from lesions in the human brainstem indicate that there are motor integration centres responsible for maintaining appropriate ocular alignment for a stable image on the macula and surrounding retina of each eye. Specific cells in the mid brain, especially in the superior colliculus of the monkey, have been demonstrated rostral to the oculomotor nucleus that respond particularly to convergence and others to divergence.[10–12]

These experimental studies are reflected clinically. The development of sensory fusion appears to parallel the development of stereopsis and may reflect maturation of the visual cortex as measured by preferential looking tests and electrophysiology.[13] Components of motor fusion also mature as sensory fusion develops. Accommodation and convergence are primitive at birth but improve over subsequent months.

The ability of the lens to increase its power is limited at birth, but improves rapidly over 6 months.[14] Simliarly, maintenance of bifoveal fixation by convergence also increases in accuracy by 6 months.[15] A further aspect of motor fusion involves the ability for bifoveal fixation, which is often developed by the age of 3 months but may continue up to 8 months.[16]

Motor arc

The lower motor neuron final common pathway for innervations of eye movements occurs via the third, fourth and sixth cranial nerves. These are equivalent to the motor neurons of the spinal cord subserving reflex movements. Defects of the efferent limbs include the lower motor neurons (third, fourth and sixth cranial nerves), the muscle endplates and the muscles themselves. Strabismus will be present in the direction of the disordered muscle movement. Binocular single vision (BSV) may only be absent in the direction of gaze of the impaired muscle movement.

Table 2.1   Actions of the extraocular muscles from primary position

Muscle	Primary	Secondary	Tertiary
Medial rectus	Adduction		
Lateral rectus	Abduction		
Inferior rectus	Depression	Excycloduction	Adduction
Superior rectus	Elevation	Incycloduction	Adduction
Inferior oblique	Excycloduction	Elevation	Abduction
Superior oblique	Incycloduction	Depression	Abduction

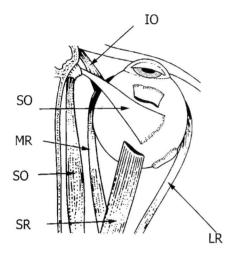

Figure 2.4   The relationship of the six extraocular muscles in the orbit. (MR = medial rectus, LR = lateral rectus, SR = superior rectus. SO = superior oblique, IO = inferior oblique)

Anatomical and physiological considerations of the motor component

Extraocular muscles

Position of the globe is maintained by seven extraocular muscles including four recti: superior, inferior, medial and lateral; two oblique muscles: superior and inferior oblique, and the levator palpebrae superioris (Figure 2.4). The lateral rectus is innervated by the sixth cranial nerve, with the superior oblique innervated by the fourth cranial nerve and the remainder by the third nerve. The four recti muscles arise from the annulus of Zinn and insert into the anterior globe in a regular fashion in the spiral of Tillaux. The superior oblique muscle arises from the orbital apex and travels along the superomedial wall of the orbit before passing through the trochlear and inserting into the posterosuperior quadrant of the globe. The inferior oblique originates from the maxilla posterior to the orbital rim and passes laterally, superiorly and posteriorly below the inferior rectus, inserting into the posterolateral part of the globe.

Positions of gaze

The primary position of gaze is where the eyes are looking straight ahead. Secondary positions of gaze include looking directly upwards, downwards, left or right and tertiary positions are the four oblique positions of up and left, up and right, down and left, down and right.

Actions of the extraocular muscles

The extraocular muscles have different actions depending on their position. Primary action is the major action of a muscle on the position of the eye in primary position. Secondary and tertiary actions are additional actions on the globe in primary position (Table 2.1).

All eye movements are rotations. The orbit, which contains the eyeball, is pyramid shaped with its medial wall in the sagittal plane. The centre of rotation of the eyeball at the front of the orbit is lateral to the origin of the recti muscles as they arise from the apex of the orbit from the sphenoid bone close to the medial wall. As a consequence of this anatomy, horizontal movements of adduction and abduction are fully subserved by the medial and lateral rectus muscles. The vertical recti differ in that they only become primarily elevators and depressors when

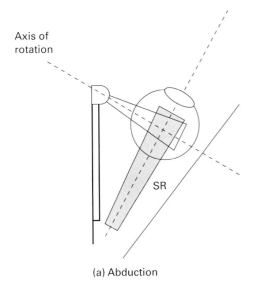

(a) Abduction

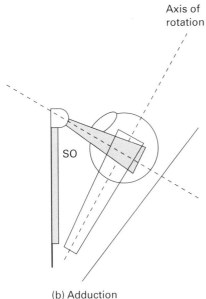

(b) Adduction

Figure 2.5 Elevation and depression of the eye is achieved in (a) abduction through the vertical recti and in (b) adduction through the obliques

the eye is abducted. When the eye is adducted, the vertical action of the superior and inferior rectus muscles diminishes, the torsional action of the recti becomes increasingly evident as the oblique muscles become the effective elevators and depressors when the eye is fully adducted (Figure 2.5). By contrast, in abduction, the ability of the superior oblique and inferior oblique muscles to elevate and depress the eye diminishes and the torsional action of the obliques becomes increasingly evident as the vertical recti again become the elevators and depressors.

Control of eye movements

Along the evolutionary scale of animals, human beings and primates have developed frontal vision and binocularity with high visual acuity. In afoveate animals, such as the rabbit, with a visual streak, eye movements are dominated by vestibular and opticokinetic stabilisation of position of the eye in space. When such animals change direction of visual attention, they must link rapid eye movement to a voluntary head movement to override the vestibular and opticokinetic influence and bring the object of interest onto the retina.[17]

With the development of frontal vision and binocular vision with high acuity of the fovea in the primate came the ability to move the eyes independently of head movements. This satisfied the need for precision of fixation as well as disjunctive or vergence movements and permitted simultaneous foveation as the object of interest was viewed at close range.[17]

In summary, vestibular, optokinetic, and fixation systems hold gaze steady in the presence of head movement so that visual images are concentrated on the retina of each eye. Saccades, smooth pursuit and vergence movements shift gaze towards a fresh object of interest and work together to hold the object of interest on each fovea (Table 2.2).

The eye muscles in primary gaze are in a constant state of tonic contraction. Whilst the final common pathways for extraocular muscle control are the cranial nerves, there are higher supranuclear centres controlling eye movements. Voluntary activity is subserved by the frontal cortex (particularly area 8) with the parieto-occipital cortex and superior colliculus serving as coordinating areas. The contribution of the cerebellum to oculomotor function is twofold:

Table 2.2   Types of eye movements and functions

Type of eye movement	Function
Vestibular	Maintains image on retina during head rotation (brief)
Optokinetic	Maintains image on retina during head rotation (sustained)
Saccade	Captures fresh objects of interest on fovea – refixation
Smooth pursuit	Maintains image of moving target on fovea – sustains fixation
Vergence	Maintains image of a single object through disjunctive movement
Visual fixation	Maintains clear visual image on the fovea with head stationary

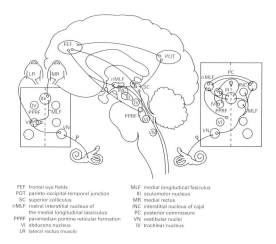

FEF   frontal eye fields
POT   parieto-occipital-temporal junction
SC   superior colliculus
riMLF   rostral interstitial nucleus of the medial longitudinal lasciculus
PPRF   paramedian pontine reticular formation
VI   abducens nucleus
LR   lateral rectus muscle
MLF   medial longitudinal fasciculus
III   oculomolor nucleus
MR   medial rectus
INC   interstitial nucleus of cajal
PC   posterior commissure
VN   vestibular nuclei
IV   trochlear nucleus

Figure 2.6   Diagram showing integrated motor control pathway for eye movement. (Reproduced with permission from Miller N in Walsh & Hoyt's Clinical Neurophthalmology)

the control of smooth pursuit eye movements through the flocculus and nodulus and the enabling of accurate refixation saccades through the dorsal vermis. There are also numerous interneuron connections between both voluntary and reflex gaze centres, mediated by pathways for horizontal gaze (PPRF, paramedian pontine reticular formation), vertical gaze (rostral interstitial nucleus of the medial longitudinal fasciculus) and vestibular systems (Figure 2.6).

The voluntary eye movements are either saccadic (fast and visually *capture* objects of visual interest) or pursuit movements (slower and used to *follow* a visual object of interest). The reflex controls add quality characteristics to the movements; for example, the influence of the cerebellum in smooth pursuit.

Most clinicians, when examining a patient, will examine the pursuit system but many omit to test the saccadic system. The slower pursuit system is examined by getting the patient to follow a specific target in the field of action of the suspected paretic muscle. This is a routine most clinicians use in testing the range of eye movement. The saccadic or refixation system is also readily examined. The patient is asked to refixate from one target to a target in the field of action of the suspected paretic muscle. The test gives an indication of the accuracy of the refixation mechanism and tests the ability to generate normal speed of a saccade. It renders

valuable information about muscle action. A weakened muscle action will manifest as a slowed saccade.

A number of terms are used in the description of eye movements. They are important to understand both in description of eye movement disorders and in an eye examination and will be briefly referred to.

- Saccades are rapid (300–700/sec) velocity refixation movements to bring objects of interest onto the macula.

- Nystagmus movements are quick phases of eye movement that occur during self-rotation. They direct the macula toward the oncoming visual experience and reset the eyes during persistent rotations. The quick phases originate in the pons and midbrain paramedian reticular formation. Phylogenetically, this is an old system and appears to share a common anatomic substrate with the more recently evolved voluntary saccadic system.

- By contrast, there are a number of slow eye movements (velocity 20–50°/sec). These include smooth pursuit that serves to hold the visual image of interest of a moving target on the centre of the macula. The parieto-occipito-temporal junction is considered an important structure in the cortical control of smooth pursuit. Associated pathways to the brainstem and cerebellum are as yet unclear. The control in this system is ipsilateral and the pathways are deep in the parietal lobe so that pure occipital lesions do not affect smooth pursuit.

- Optokinetic movements serve to hold images of the visual environment steady on the centre of the macula during sustained head rotation. We previously referred to disturbance of optokinetic nystagmus (OKN) in failure to develop binocular vision. Pure OKN consists of a slow phase following the stripes on an OKN drum interspersed with saccades to refixate oncoming stripes.

- Vestibular movement, namely in the vestibulo-ocular reflex, holds images of the visual world during sustained head rotation. Vestibular eye movements are based on the labyrinthine-pontine pathways and take information from the ampullae of the semi-circular canals to generate these ocular movements.

- Vergence via the occipito-mesencephalic pathway is a disconjugate eye movement enabling bifoveal fixation during convergence.

References

1. Corbetta M, Miezin FM, Dobmeyer S, Shulman GL, Petersen SE. Selective and divided attention during visual discriminations of shape, color, and speed: functional anatomy by positron emission tomography. *J Neurosci* 1991;**11**:2383–402.

2. Dobson V, Teller DY. Visual acuity in human infants: a review and comparison of behavioral and electrophysiological studies. *Vision Res* 1978;**18**:1469–83.

3. Norcia AM, Tyler CW, Allen D. Electrophysiological assessment of contrast sensitivity in human infants. *Am J Optom Physiol Optics* 1986;**63**:12–15.

4. Hubel DH, Wiesel TN. Binocular interaction in striate cortex of kittens reared with artificial squint. *J Neurophysiol* 1965;**28**:1041–59.

5. Shimojo S. Pre-stereoptic binocular vision in infants. *Vision Res* 1986;**26**:501.

6. Gwiazda JB, Held R. Binocular function in human infants: correlation of stereoptic and fusion rivalry discrimination. *J Pediatr Ophthalmol Strabismus* 1989;**26**:128.

7. Norcia AM, Sutter EE, Tyler CW. Electrophysiological evidence of the existence of coarse and fine disparity mechanisms in humans. *Vision Res* 1985;**25**:1603–11.

8. Held R, Birch E, Gwiazda J. Stereoacuity of human infants. *Proc Natl Acad Sci USA* 1980;**77**:5572–4.

9. Naegele JH. The postnatal development of monocular optokinetic nystagmus in infants. *Vision Res* 1982;**22**:341.

10. Mays LP, Gamlin PD, Tello CA. Neural control of vergence eye movements: neurons encoding vergence velocity. *J Neurophysiol* 1986;**56**:1007–21.

11. Mays L. Neural control of vergence eye movements: convergence and divergence neurons in the midbrain. *J Neurophysiol* 1984;**51**:1091–107.

12. Judge SC. Neurons in the monkey midbrain with activity related to vergence. *J Neurophysiol* 1986;**55**:915–29.

13. Birch E, Shimojo S, Held R. Preferential looking assessment of fusion and stereopsis in infants aged 1–6 months. *Invest Ophthalmol Vis Sci* 1991;**32**:820.

14. Brookman KE. Ocular accommodation in human infants. *Am J Optom Physiol Optics* 1983;**60**:91–9.

15. Aslin RN. Development of binocular fixation in human infants. *Am J Optom Physiol Optics* 1977;**23**:133–50.

16. Archer SM, Sondhi N, Helveston EM. Strabismus in infancy. *Ophthalmology* 1989;**96**:133–7.

17. Leigh RJ, Zee DS. The properties and neural substrate of eye movements. In: Leigh RJ, Zee DS, eds. *The Neurology of Eye Movements*. Philadelphia: FA Davis, 1991.

3 Consequences of breakdown of binocular vision

Introduction

Vision develops with a definite chronology and integration with other sensory inputs to the developing central nervous system. This development takes place dramatically in the first 4 years, but does not approach maturity until the end of the first decade of life. Breakdown of binocular vision has different sequelae depending on the age of onset, reflecting the maturity of the visual system. Consequences of breakdown in children before the visual system matures may include an alternating strabismus, or a strabismus with fixation preference for one eye. Because of the plasticity of the developing brain, amblyopia and the adaptations of suppression and anomalous retinal correspondence occur and diplopia and visual confusion are avoided.[1] This is in contrast to the older patient with breakdown of normal binocular vision, who may suffer from diplopia and visual confusion as long as there is vision in both eyes, although she may also learn to suppress the image from one eye.[2]

Sequelae of strabismus in the immature visual system (children)

Amblyopia

The period of development in which experience plays an influential role has been termed the critical period.[3] The plasticity of the central nervous system necessary for this development is associated in the maturing visual system with the need for clear imaging on the fovea of each eye. In turn, this is associated with retinal rivalry between each eye such that if the clarity of the image in the fovea in one eye is disturbed, vision in the better eye will be reinforced. If the poor vision leads to strabismus in that eye, the loss of vision may be compounded by strabismic amblyopia (amblyopia that is secondary to the shift of the object of regard away from the fovea of the squinting eye). The lack of clarity of the image on the fovea may be due to a media obstruction such as a partial cataract, or may be due to a difference between the two eyes associated with difference in the axial measurements of the two eyes, so-called anisometropic amblyopia. The critical period for pattern deprivation amblyopia to occur and be reversed completely in the human eye is estimated to be in the first 3 months after birth, whereas the critical period for strabismic amblyopia is thought to be up to 5–6 years of age and anisometropic amblyopia up to 7–8 years. The significance of these timeframes is only as a guide and will vary depending on a number of factors, for example density of a cataract, the degree of anisometropia, or whether there is a combination with other forms of amblyopia (see amblyopia in Chapters 1 and 7).

Retinal correspondence and ARC

Points on the retina of each eye that share a common subjective visual direction are said to be corresponding. An object is then perceived to

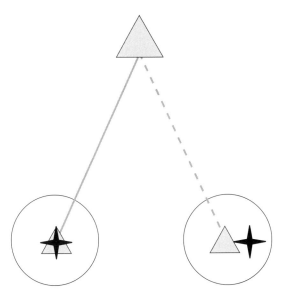

Figure 3.1 Anomalous retinal correspondence (ARC). ARC occurs when the fovea (black cross) of the fixing eye is paired with a non-foveal point of the fellow eye so that they acquire a common visual direction in order to visualise an object (red triangle). The fovea of the non-fixing eye is suppressed

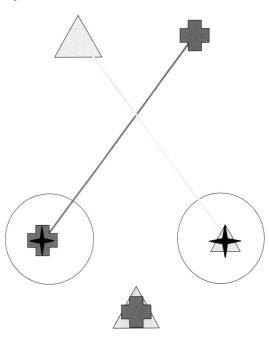

Figure 3.2 If corresponding points, for example, each macula (black cross), are simultaneously stimulated by different objects (triangle and dark grey cross), confusion may arise

be coming from the same direction in space. Normal retinal correspondence occurs if each of these points on each retina has the same spatial relationship with the fovea of each eye. Anomalous retinal correspondence (ARC) occurs if there is a different spatial relationship between these points and the foveas in each eye; this may be a consequence of long-standing ocular deviation in children (Figure 3.1).

Sequelae of strabismus in the mature visual system (adults)

Visual confusion

Visual confusion arises from simultaneous fovea-dominated perception of two different images superimposed upon each other, as in the presence of ocular misalignment. Objects that are separated in real space are perceived to belong to the same location in subjective space. Visual confusion is associated with ocular

misalignment, is transient in children and more likely to be seen in the adult (Figure 3.2).

Diplopia

Diplopia or double vision occurs when an image simultaneously falls on the fovea of one eye and a non-foveal point on the fellow eye, usually from ocular misalignment. The same object is seen as having two different locations in subjective space, with the foveal image clearer than the non-foveal image. Diplopia may result in suppression in the younger patient (Figure 3.3).

"Horror fusionis" is an intractable form of diplopia where there is both a loss of ability to maintain fusion and an absence of suppression; this may occur after head injuries, surgical correction of monocular cataract in adults with previous suppression, or after prolonged

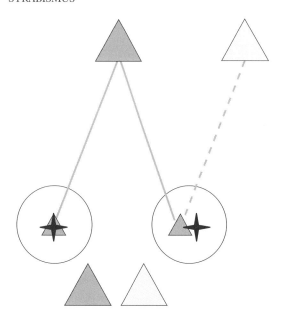

Figure 3.3 Diplopia arises from simultaneous appreciation of two different images of the one object due to loss of binocular vision. It arises because the image (dark grey triangle) in the non-fixing eye falls on a location outside the macula (black cross) and is projected to a different point in space. The image in the non-fixing eye is more faint than that in the fixing eye

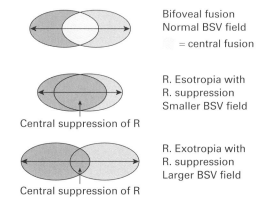

Bifoveal fusion
Normal BSV field

= central fusion

R. Esotropia with
R. suppression
Smaller BSV field

Central suppression of R

R. Exotropia with
R. suppression
Larger BSV field

Central suppression of R

Figure 3.4 Fields of binocular vision and suppression. Note: (i) In normal binocular vision there is central fusion. The peripheral temporal field of each eye has no overlap from the other eye, is monocular, is not suppressed, and contributes to the binocular field, even in the presence of strabismus. (ii) The double arrow-head represents the width of the binocular field of vision, being smaller in esotropia than in exotropia

disruption of fusion. In severe head injury with bilateral superior oblique palsy, the inability to fuse may be caused by the excyclotropia, usually of more than 10°.

Suppression

Suppression is a mechanism which eliminates visual confusion and diplopia by removing an unwanted image. It may also eliminate fusion and stereopsis in the mature visual system in the adult, for example in long-standing unilateral cataract. The suppression scotoma is roughly 2·5° in diameter[4] and differs in size and shape in strabismus patients with exotropias compared to esotropias.[5] The extreme peripheral temporal field of each eye has no overlap with the other eye, is monocular, is not suppressed in amblyopia and contributes to the extent of the visual field (Figure 3.4). Suppression may also occur in the adult as a result of an adaptation to visual confusion.

Suppression develops in the immature visual cortex as a response to differing inputs from each eye and is a barrier to the development of fusion. In the immature visual system its presence can eradicate the fusion and stereopsis that have already developed. The whole of the visual field of the deviating eye is suppressed. The overlap with the visual field of the fixing eye is suppressed and the remainder of the visual field of the deviating eye is not suppressed.[6] The binocular field is wider in an exotropic patient as a consequence and smaller in an esotropic patient (Figure 3.4).

Suppression is an important aspect to consider in surgery. If there is suppression of the retina there is no diplopia; however, if surgery overcorrects the strabismus, diplopia may be evoked. In the visually immature child, suppression will develop in response to the new eye position, but in the visually mature adult, diplopia may persist and be troublesome.

Significance of strabismus with loss of fusion in the adult

The majority of sudden onset strabismus in adults occurs in a mature visual system. Diplopia is a constant manifestation of strabismus in these circumstances. It carries with it essential adaptations resulting from suppression. The presentation of loss of binocular vision is usually primarily a motor rather than a sensory problem. Inability to fuse may be caused by central fusion loss. In an adult patient who complains of diplopia, where there is evidence of loss of central fusion an underlying organic cause should be excluded, including the possibility of an intracranial tumour.

Decompensation may occur in the adult who has a compensated developmental strabismus. A typical case is the development of strabismus in a case of fourth nerve palsy with binocular vision, which has been previously compensated by abnormal head posture. Evidence of the long-standing nature of such a case might be gained from photos of abnormal head posture, which, at the same time, demonstrate in the adult the presence of larger fusion amplitudes than normal. Breakdown of binocular vision in the adult in such cases is often based upon fatigue of motor control. Long-standing sensory adaptations tend to remain stable. An exception is the occasional spontaneous loss of suppression (for example in a long-standing adult esotropia), leading to double vision. It may develop with trauma or emotional stress.

Relevant clinical conclusions

Normal binocular vision (NBV), if incomplete in infancy, develops with fusion and stereopsis by age 5–10 years. In the first 3 months of life superimposing of visual images occurs. At 3 months evidence of binocular fusion is seen in rivalry aversion. Between the ages of 3–6 months sensitivity to stereoscopic disparities improves.[7] Stereoscopic development of vision may continue to develop until 8 or 9 years of age.[8] It follows that surgical restoration of ocular alignment before the age of 2 offers a greater chance of binocular vision.[9–12] Whether even earlier surgery results in more superior degrees of binocularity is under investigation. Normally the initial primitive temporonasal visual pursuit movement is replaced by symmetric nasotemporal pursuit if normal binocular vision develops. This can usually be demonstrated with the OKN (opticokinetic nystagmus) stripe or drum by 3–5 months.[13] In congenital (infantile) esotropia, eye misalignment usually occurs after age 3–4 months, indicating some opportunity for binocular M-neuron development prior to the development of the strabismus. Maturation of NBV is associated with maturation of visual functions. The earlier the barrier to maturation occurs, the more easily normal binocular visual development is disrupted.

Clinically one can demonstrate normal binocular vision after 3–5 months using a 15 D base out prism. As the infant views the target, the eye without the prism maintains fixation and the eye with the prism makes a convergent movement to also take up fixation and maintain fusion. Before 3–5 months it is not uncommon to see variable angles of divergent eye movement and incomitant eye movement.[14] There is therefore a critical period spanning 3–5 months after birth during which the binocular neuronal connections in the M stream of the visual cortex provide signals for normal binocular alignment of the eyes. The normal development of the sensory aspect of binocular vision M-neuron connections by the age of 6 months is essential for the development of fusional eye movements in an orderly way.

Three important clinical points to emphasise.

- Firstly, small angle strabismus, particularly divergence in the first 3 months, is so frequent as to be regarded as normal maturation, and should not be diagnosed as a squint but the child should be followed if there is any doubt.

- Secondly, in the binocular testing of conjugate movement in the first 3 months of life, it is not uncommon to see pursuit as a series of micro-saccades and the pursuit system not smooth.

- Finally, infants who fail to develop normal binocular vision will be found to have a latent fixation nystagmus because of failure to develop the normal nasotemporal pursuit. The eyes tend to drift nasally and show fast phase corrective jerks and the nystagmus increases if one eye is covered, which is why this clinical finding is described as latent nystagmus. The observation requires a visually attentive child and careful observation by the clinician. Any disturbance of clear imaging of visual targets sufficient to interrupt the development of normal binocular vision in the first 6 months of life will be accompanied by a similar nystagmus. It is not confined to congenital infantile esotropia.

In congenital infantile esotropia (see Chapter 4) during the first 6 months, there is failure to establish normal M-neuron connections required for normal nasotemporal pursuit and pursuit asymmetry persists.[15] For this reason when pursuit asymmetry is present in an adult, it indicates that strabismus since infancy is likely and suggests the possibility that the presence of subnormal vision may be strabismic amblyopia. The association of amblyopia with disruption of normal binocular vision is more likely to occur under the age of 5 or 6 years. Adult patients may develop strabismus from loss of fusion due to persistent visual deprivation but they do not develop amblyopia.

Clinically, it is important to understand eye movements in the first months of life particularly if one examines the eyes monocularly. The infant responds to the information contained in the M (magnocellular) pathway, showing preference to targets that move in a temporal to nasal direction in the visual field. By contrast, the infant tracks targets poorly that move

temporally with regard to the eye being tested.[13] The difference relates to movement response to visual stimulus, not the motor pathway.[15] After 3–5 months this nasal bias of visual pursuit is replaced by symmetrical nasotemporal pursuit if normal binocular vision develops. The development of high visual acuity after birth depends on maturation of synaptic connections, the visual path and primary visual cortex. The development of normal binocular vision requires an equal visual input to the visual cortex from each eye and during development there is a competition between the eyes for representation within the visual cortex. With a balanced input there would be an associated matching neuronal connectivity of the information processed from each eye and the possibility of normal binocular vision. Therefore a deficit of the visual image from one of the eyes results in altered neuronal connectivity and the possibility of breakdown of binocular vision. Specific clinical examples include variants of Ciancia syndrome and strabismus associated with congenital cataract.

Specific clinical examples

Variants of Ciancia syndrome

With malformation of one eye, such as severe microphthalmos or surgically induced prenatal absence of one eye in an animal model, permanent changes can be demonstrated in the cellular organisation and synaptic connectivity in the areas of the brain subserving binocular vision.[16] The lateral geniculate nucleus has an absence of representation of the eye removed and additional connections are formed between the intact eye and the geniculate neurons that have lost their input. In the visual cortex ocular dominance columns fail to develop. The frequent result is an abducting nystagmus in the sound eye with a null point in convergence reminiscent of that seen in Ciancia syndrome with face turn away from the microphthalmic or defective eye.

Strabismus associated with congenital cataract

With unilateral or asymmetrical congenital cataract in the first weeks of life, there is urgent need to have clear imaging with optical correction. Delay until 4–5 months means poor input from the low-resolution M neurons subserving the affected eye. Even with surgery for unilateral congenital cataract in the first or second days of life, it is difficult to achieve optimal optical correction because of myopic shift with growth of the eye, and the absence of flexible accommodation in the operated eye prejudices the operated eye in favour of the unoperated eye with increased risk of amblyopia. Evidence from clinical and basic science studies suggests that when there is frustration of normal M-neuron connections, there is a likelihood of failure of the later development of the higher resolution parvocellular system and greater likelihood of strabismus. The eyes must be aligned early and receive sharply focused images for M neurons to develop normally with nasotemporal motion sensitivity and stereopsis. Some occlusion of the unoperated eye may be important to assist this. However, total occlusion throughout the waking hours of the infant would frustrate this.

Absence of fusion

Absence of fusion may reflect a hereditary defect in the quality of binocular single vision (BSV). In rare cases it can also follow injury. Secondary loss of BSV particularly due to injury is sometimes known as "horror fusionis". It may follow a long period of disrupted binocular vision as seen in a long-standing unilateral cataract in an adult. Restoration of sight following surgery in such cases may result in intractable diplopia because of the loss of fusion ability. In a child or adult presenting with sudden onset strabismus with diplopia and loss of binocular vision with absent fusion, cerebral tumour should be suspected and excluded.

Whether binocular vision is a learned function or inherent and innate within the organisation of the visual system is an unresolved debate. The view that binocular vision has been acquired phylogenetically rather than ontogenetically is supported by the fact that within families, children with strabismus may have siblings whose binocular vision is deficient even though the siblings do not have strabismus. The work of Hubel and Wiesel is also supportive of this view. It includes the fact that binocular vision and spatial orientation cannot be improved with experience and training.

References

1. Burian HM. The sensorial retinal relationships in comitant strabismus. *Arch Ophthalmol* 1947;**37**:336–40.
2. Billson FA, Fitzgerald BA, Provis JM. Visual deprivation in infancy and childhood: clinical aspects. *Aust NZ J Ophthalmol* 1985;**13**:279–86.
3. Hubel DH, Livingstone MS. Segregation of form, colour and stereopsis in primate area 18. *J Neurosci* 1987;7:3378–415.
4. Tychsen L. Binocular vision. In: Hart WM, ed. *Adler's Physiology of the Eye*. St Louis: Mosby, 1992:773.
5. Jampolsky A. Characteristics of suppression in strabismus. *Arch Ophthalmol* 1955;**54**:683–9.
6. Pratt-Johnson JA, Tillson G. Unilateral congenital cataract: binocular status after treatment. *J Pediatr Ophthalmol Strabismus* 1989;**26**:72–4.
7. Held R, Birch E, Gwiazda J. Stereoacuity of human infants. *Proc Natl Acad Sci USA* 1980;**77**:5572–4.
8. Romano PE, Romano JA, Puklin JE. Stereoacuity development in children with normal binocular single vision. *Am J Ophthalmol* 1975;**79**:966–71.
9. Corbetta M, Miezin FM, Dobmeyer S, Shulman GL, Petersen SE. Selective and divided attention during visual discriminations of shape, color, and speed: functional anatomy by positron emission tomography. *J Neurosci* 1991;**11**:2383–402.
10. Lennie P. Parallel visual pathways: a review. *Vision Res* 1980;**20**:561–94.
11. Stone J, Dreher B, Leventhal A. Hierarchical and parallel mechanisms in the organization of visual cortex. *Brain Res* 1979;**180**:345–94.
12. Zeki SM. Functional specialisation in the visual cortex of the rhesus monkey. *Nature* 1978;**274**:423–8.
13. Naegele JH. The postnatal development of monocular optokinetic nystagmus in infants. *Vision Res* 1982;**22**:341.
14. Nixon R. Incidence of strabismus in neonates. *Am J Ophthalmol* 1985;**100**:798.
15. Tychsen L, Hurtig RR, Scott WE. Pursuit is impaired but the vestibulo-ocular reflex is normal in infantile strabismus. *Arch Ophthalmol* 1985;**103**:536–9.
16. Horton J. The central visual pathways. In: Hart WM, ed. *Adler's Physiology of the Eye: Clinical Applications*. St Louis: Mosby, 1992.

Section II
Strabismus in the decades of life

Overview of Section II

Consideration of strabismus in the decades of life is important for two reasons.

- It draws attention to the fact that earlier in life, the causes are likely to be developmental in origin, whereas in adult years tumours, thyroid eye disease, trauma, and myasthenia gravis are more common, culminating in the older adult where vascular disease is more dominant.

- It highlights in the child the consequences of strabismus in an immature visual system as distinct from the adolescent and adult where breakdown of binocular single vision occurs in a mature visual system.

Nevertheless, it is important for the clinician to realise that because strabismus is common in childhood, a significant part of adult eye movement disorders may present with residua of childhood onset strabismus.

In the first decade (0–10 years) of infancy and childhood

In the first decade of life the majority of cases of strabismus have non-progressive underlying pathology or a static neurological abnormality. However, strabismus in the first decade also has added complexity because of the secondary consequence of amblyopia. The earlier the onset, the more likely the strabismus will be manifest without any obvious underaction of ocular muscle movements, although vertical muscle imbalance may present later with disturbance of action of the oblique muscles or vertical rectus muscles. Craniofacial anomalies or inappropriate milestones should alert the clinician to the possibility of associated pathology as the basis of strabismus.

In the second decade (10–20 years)

In the second and succeeding decades of life the strabismus is increasingly likely to affect specific third, fourth or sixth cranial nerve dysfunction. In adolescence and early adult life refractive changes in the eye are occurring and it is also important to be alert to clinical conditions that may underlie strabismus, including trauma and benign intracranial hypertension.

In the third, fourth, and fifth decades (20–50 years)

Trauma, thyroid eye disease, multiple sclerosis, myasthenia gravis, developmental vascular anomalies including berry aneurysms and neoplasms need to be considered. Other inflammatory conditions including sarcoidosis, infectious polyneuritis, myositis, orbital pseudo tumour and otitis media are important causes of strabismus within this age group.

Succeeding decades (50–80 years)

Degenerative vascular disease, hypertension, diabetes mellitus, carotid cavernous fistula, both direct and indirect (dural shunts) will be more frequent causes for breakdown of binocular vision. Vascular syndromes in this age group and cerebral tumours are common causes for strabismus in the older adult.

4 Childhood onset of strabismus

Childhood strabismus is distinguished by the risk of amblyopia. The strabismus may be considered in the context of a number of syndromes; those that are predominantly horizontal (concomitant) and without marked movement deficits and those that are incomitant with more exaggerated movement deficits. Both concomitant and incomitant strabismus may be associated with vertical muscle imbalance at presentation. Concomitant horizontal deviations may develop vertical deviations later with characteristic alphabet patterns and need to be followed carefully in order to obtain optimal outcomes. These are most commonly seen in congenital (infantile) esotropia and for completeness' sake will be discussed with this entity.

Amblyopia

Recognition and treatment of amblyopia is a fundamental component of management of strabismus. Principles of management are essentially directed at early detection and treatment to produce equal vision, only then followed by strabismus surgery aimed at ocular alignment. Assessment and management of amblyopia are further discussed in Chapters 6 and 7. The basic science which underpins clinical manifestations of amblyopia is discussed in Chapter 1. Various forms of amblyopia may be present in strabismus cases; for example, there may be a combination of strabismic and pattern deprivation amblyopia due to a unilateral cataract or refractive cause.

Types of amblyopia

Strabismic amblyopia

Strabismic amblyopia is unilateral. It occurs less frequently in untreated congenital infantile esotropias (20%) compared with acquired infantile esotropias (100%).[1] Intermittent exotropias, on the other hand, usually do not produce strabismic amblyopia, as there is fusion at near fixation.

Refractive amblyopia

Refractive amblyopia caused by uncorrected ametropia may be unilateral or bilateral and may involve a meridional component from astigmatism. Anisometropic amblyopia may occur if the refractive error is unilateral and may be associated with strabismus in approximately 30% of cases. Aniseikonia from correction of a large difference in refractive error appears to be tolerated better in children than adults, and should not be used as an excuse not to offer glasses and occlusion.[2]

Pattern deprivation amblyopia

The absence of patterned visual stimulation of the fovea during the first few months of life is particularly devastating. It is important to recognise that amblyopia may occur as a result of a media opacity such as congenital cataract, corneal scar, retinoblastoma or vitreous haemorrhage. Pattern deprivation amblyopia may be unilateral or bilateral and may be associated with strabismus if unilateral.

Iatrogenic deprivation amblyopia

The treatment of an ocular condition such as an eyelid lesion or corneal ulcer with an occluding eye patch may also result in deprivation amblyopia, especially in the first weeks of life. Occlusion may be safe if not used for more than 80% of the waking day. In a unilateral dense cataract at birth or bilateral dense cataract at birth requiring surgery, bilateral occlusion in the early weeks of life may prolong the critical period. This allows more time to achieve equal imaging in both eyes and reduce the risk of amblyopia.

"Concomitant" strabismus

Congenital esotropia syndromes

Esotropia in childhood is the commonest form of strabismus seen amongst Caucasians in clinical practice. It represents more than half the ocular deviations in childhood (Figure 4.1). With a presentation of esotropia under the age of 3 months, a motor imbalance will persist and be seen as an associated latent nystagmus with defective nasotemporal optokinetic nystagmus (see Section I).

Concomitant esotropia in infancy includes congenital (infantile) esotropia, which needs to be identified and separated clinically from Ciancia syndrome (esotropia with abduction nystagmus, nystagmus compensation syndrome) and refractive accommodative esotropia. Esotropias associated with neurological abnormalities also need to be identified. Finally, in cases with poor vision at birth, particularly microphthalmia with poor vision in one eye (sensory strabismus), the eye with good vision may behave like Ciancia syndrome with abducting nystagmus and compensatory head posture.

Congenital (infantile) esotropia has been referred to as either infantile esotropia or essential esotropia. The term congenital esotropia is used in this text. The esotropia is not always present at birth although the underlying causative mechanism may be. This is a condition that

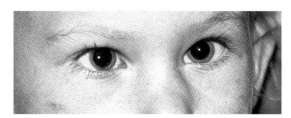

Figure 4.1   Congenital esotropia

affects as many as 2% of children in the population, although the incidence may be declining. The cause of infantile esotropia is largely unknown. There are risk factors for infantile esotropia, including family history and *in utero* drug exposure – particularly exposure to smoking. Extreme prematurity and children with identifiable neurologic injury, for example perinatal hypoxia–ischaemia, are also at higher risk for esotropia. Other neurological syndromes such as hydrocephalus and Arnold–Chiari syndrome also may cause strabismus identical to congenital esotropia in the first year of life. However, the clinical neurological abnormality may not be recognised early, emphasising the need for caution for early surgery in the first year of life.

Clinical features

The typical presentation is a child who seems to have straight eyes for the first 2 or 3 months of life and then rather suddenly develops a large angle esotropia. The typical angle of deviation is from 45 to 60 prism dioptres and the pattern is usually comitant. In some situations an A or V pattern may become apparent, although in the first year of life A and V patterns are usually not easily recognised. There is seldom any significant refractive error (for example, hyperopia) greater than 2·0 dioptres. Many children with infantile esotropia cross-fixate, converging either eye to observe the contralateral field. As a consequence they may appear to have bilateral sixth nerve palsies. A trial of uniocular patching will readily demonstrate full ocular movement. Cross-fixation indicates that either eye is used equally well and they do not have amblyopia.

Congenital esotropia never develops later than 6 months of age and more often develops at 2–3 months. In addition, the syndrome in many cases includes primary inferior oblique overaction with a V pattern of movement, dissociated vertical deviation (DVD), nystagmus and occasionally nystagmus compensation syndrome. Most of these additional features may not be apparent in the first year of life. Rarely, an A pattern, often in association with superior oblique overaction, is seen. Because of the failure to develop normal binocular vision, asymmetrical optokinetic nystagmus (OKN) will be present.

In the untreated case of congenital esotropia, both eyes may be esotropic and abduction is limited in each eye. Typically, cross-fixation with the convergent eye is used to observe the opposite visual field, but this changes as the child grows and by 2 years of age, they will look with one eye straight ahead and the other eye convergent. In congenital esotropia, inferior oblique overaction is not usually present in the first months but appears before the age of 2 in up to 78% of patients.[3] Dissociated vertical deviation (DVD) tends to occur later in up to 70% of cases by 18 months to 3 years. An abnormal head posture or face turn may occur if nystagmus is present. There is a suggestion that the incidence of amblyopia may be less for untreated cases.[1,4,20] The natural history of the untreated case is reviewed in Chapter 5.

Management

Management of congenital esotropia involves occlusion to ensure equal vision and the systematic correction of the associated features, which are part of the natural history of the disease. Though not present at diagnosis, they should be discussed with the parents as they may appear later. Assessment and therapies are discussed in Section III.

Cross-fixation implies equal vision. When unilateral fixation preference does occur this requires treatment for amblyopia (particularly in Ciancia syndrome or cases with asymmetrising factors). Preference for cross-fixation may be confused with deficient abduction. A short period of occlusion of each eye, for example half an hour a day, will readily demonstrate that the child has full abduction and no preference for fixing either eye. The family in the home situation may manage occlusion.

Large angle esotropia should be measured in prism dioptres at distance. With cross-fixation and no occlusion the convergent angle is likely to increase. These cases often come to surgery. It is important to measure the deviation especially in the week before surgery. If the esotropia is more than 45–50 dioptres the deviation will not be corrected with glasses. However, post surgery glasses are often useful in correcting residual deviation.

Surgical alignment before the age of 2 years increases the quality of binocular vision but there is no convincing evidence that alignment before the age of 12 months results in increased binocularity[5] (see Section III for further details). Surgical correction of esotropia may also result in an increased binocular field from inclusion of the overlapping temporal field segments.[6]

Follow up

Untreated patients with large angle squints generally will maintain equal vision (6/6) alternating suppression and no fusion, although amblyopia is a risk if they do not alternate. Ocular alignment under the age of 3 needs careful follow up because small angle squint is associated with a higher incidence of amblyopia.[1]

Associated features of congenital esotropia

Dissociated vertical deviation   The basis of dissociated vertical deviation is not understood. Dissociated vertical deviation occurs in more than half the patients with congenital esotropia syndrome.[7,8] The parents of a child with DVD will report that one eye or alternately either eye will intermittently elevate and appear to move

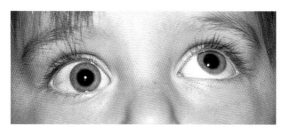

Figure 4.2 Dissociated vertical deviation (DVD) is a recognised association of congenital esotropia. It is clinically distinguished from an overacting inferior oblique by the absence of a V pattern of movement. However, both DVD and esotropia may occur together in congenital esotropia and present a diagnostic challenge

outward. This is due to the affected eye elevating and undergoing excyclotorsion. This feature may be demonstrated in the clinic by observing under cover. When the cover is removed the eye may come down with incyclotorsion, returning to the same position as before the cover dissociated the eyes. DVD is not associated with hypotropia of the other eye even when it appears unilateral. The eye is not associated with a V pattern of movement when the eyes observe a distant target with chin down as opposed to the neck extended (Figure 4.2).

In congenital esotropia it is important to distinguish between vertical deviation due to inferior oblique overaction or DVD. This may be difficult as both conditions may be present. Primary inferior oblique overaction should not be diagnosed in the absence of a V pattern of movement. Furthermore, when the patient is tested in the field of action of the inferior oblique, and the patient has inferior oblique overaction, the non-fixing eye will be hypotropic and when the fixing eye is covered, the lower eye will move up.

Inferior oblique overaction may be associated with a strictly unilateral superior oblique paresis. This will be associated with hypotropia when fixing with the unaffected eye, which is increased when the head is tilted to the same side (Bielschowsky head tilt test – see Chapter 6). The

increase of hypotropia also occurs with conjugate gaze to the opposite side in the field of action of the inferior oblique overacting antagonist muscle.

Primary overaction of the inferior oblique Primary overaction of the inferior oblique is seen as part of the congenital esotropic syndrome in some 30% of cases. The disturbance in the pattern of movement as a result of inferior oblique overaction is a V pattern of movement. In addition, some apparent weakness of the superior oblique is frequently seen. Where there is weakness of the superior oblique, the overaction of the ipsilateral inferior oblique is readily understood. The term primary inferior oblique overaction is used because the underaction of the superior oblique is not always present. It is important to confirm the associated V pattern or A pattern, as these may be important causes for a variable strabismic angle. The V pattern of eye movement is by far the most common pattern whilst esotropia associated with A pattern is rarely observed (Figure 4.3).

In testing inferior oblique overaction, it is important to control accommodation. This is assisted if refractive error is corrected and the child's eye movements are examined at distance. With the child maintaining fixation, the clinician may elevate and lower the chin, taking measurement of the ocular deviation and comparing the deviation measured in the elevated and depressed positions. It may show some 25 dioptres of difference in the angle measured in the V syndrome. The overaction of the inferior oblique should be verified by the Parks 3-step test and the Bielschowsky head tilt test for fourth nerve palsy. Absence of a V pattern of movement raises doubts about the diagnosis of overaction of the inferior oblique.

Latent nystagmus and nystagmus blockage syndrome (Ciancia) syndrome Latent nystagmus is a common association of congenital esotropia. With occlusion of one eye the latent nystagmus will become manifest. The

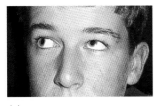

(a)

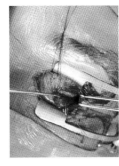

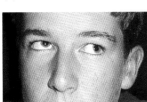

(b)

(c)

Figure 4.3   Bilteral inferior oblique overaction in a young man (a, b) with an enlarged inferior oblique muscle found at surgery (c). Confirmation of the diagnosis is based upon presence of a V pattern and enlarged inferior oblique muscle on exploration of the muscle. DVD may also be misdiagnosed and is often not associated with a V pattern although may be present

majority of cases of congenital esotropia syndrome will have latent nystagmus, that is, nystagmus observed under cover and in the fixing eye. This may be manifest as a small amplitude nystagmus that may be associated with a head turn so that the fixing eye is adducted. If the child has no preference with either eye in congenital esotropia syndrome the head posture may alternate with the face turned toward the side of the eye that is fixing and convergent.

Ciancia syndrome is the association of congenital esotropia with head turn to compensate for nystagmus. In this syndrome asymmetrical OKN will be present. Induced OKN reveals a normal response to the target moving from the temporal to nasal field but an abnormal response to the target moving from the nasal to temporal field. The persistence of this primitive response usually indicates a poor prognosis for binocular vision.

This syndrome, also referred to as nystagmus blockage syndrome, is another example of nystagmus with a null point, with the difference that the null point is in a position of convergence. Ciancia syndrome has all the appearance of infantile esotropia, with the exception that, when the eye abducts, a type of nystagmus occurs in the infant. There is a face turn usually marked with the fixing eye in adduction. These children may cross-fixate and therefore make large head turns to the left or to the right, depending on which eye they prefer to use at the time.

Management of nystagmus blockage syndrome is similar to that of infantile esotropia. However, Ciancia syndrome generally requires a larger amount of strabismus surgery and the effect of this may be to eliminate the abduction nystagmus altogether.[9] The abnormal head posture is often only obvious when detailed material is being studied. In children there may be difficulty in the classroom seeing the blackboard. The child should sit on the side of the classroom to which the face turn is directed.

Differential diagnosis of congenital esotropia syndrome

It is important to consider the differential diagnoses in this syndrome. There is a need to exclude a monocular sensory deficit, as may occur with structural damage to the macula and the retina, for example in retinoblastoma.

Duane syndrome and Moebius syndrome are important oculomotor disorders to recognise. In Duane syndrome, there is non-comitancy of the strabismus pattern with an abduction deficit and enophthalmos on abduction. Moebius syndrome may also present as an esotropia but with obvious abduction deficits and bilateral facial nerve paresis.

Parents need to be informed that the management of infantile esotropia does not end with ocular alignment and that treatment with occlusion remains an important part of management until the child's visual system is mature. The large angle with cross-fixation and with no amblyopia, once converted to a very small angle strabismus problem, is much more likely to develop a fixation preference for one eye or the other, allowing the fellow eye then to develop amblyopia. Still, surgical correction remains the mainstay of treatment and offers the best possibility of a form of binocular vision and a stable alignment. In some centres, botulinum toxin is used and optical correction either before or occasionally after strabismus surgery may be helpful, but these have not been demonstrated conclusively to offer any particular advantages in terms of the quality of binocular vision available as compared with surgical alignment.

Accommodative esotropia

The most common cause of strabismus in the first 5 years of life is accommodative esotropia. In the near reflex there is a relatively precise ratio of convergence of the eyes to units of accommodation. Children who have more convergence per unit of accommodation than required will develop a breakdown of their fusion mechanism and develop acquired accommodative esotropia.

Despite the later onset of accommodative esotropia when compared to infantile esotropia, amblyopia is more common in accommodative esotropia. Many children will have an asymmetric refractive error, with one eye being more hyperopic or more astigmatic than the other. High accommodative convergence to accommodation ratios (AC:A ratios) may also occur. In this situation, an esotropia that is greater for near fixation than distance fixation will occur. More rarely, this AC:A ratio may be affected to the point that a child will have an exotropia for distance fixation and esotropia for near fixation.

Unlike congenital (infantile) esotropias, where refractive error is not marked and onset is less than 6 months, accommodative esotropia has onset between 6 and 12 months, although rare cases do occur in infancy. Infants with congenital (infantile) esotropia with hypermetropia more than +3 D demand a trial of spectacle correction. For refractive errors less than +3 D, this will

rarely affect the decision for strabismus surgery, though the spectacle correction may be of value post-operatively.

Children with poor vision in one eye including retinoblastoma or microphthalmos may be convergent or divergent. However, a number of cases with poor vision in one eye at birth will develop a clinical picture reminiscent of Ciancia syndrome.[10]

Management

The management of this condition understandably should target accommodation. Once accommodation or the need to accommodate to focus clearly is eliminated, the convergent squint often disappears. Therefore, children with accommodative esotropia are carefully refracted and any refractive error of any significance is corrected. Since this is usually a hyperopic refractive error, hyperopic spectacles are the mainstay of treatment. With early diagnosis, approximately two thirds of children with accommodative esotropia can expect to experience good ocular alignment. However, about one third require surgical management with re-operations occasionally necessary. As in infantile esotropia, oblique muscle overaction is known to occur and may also require further management.

Acquired esotropias in children

Children developing esotropia within the first 6 months of life are defined as having congenital esotropia. Those developing esotropia between 18 months and 3 years, having straight eyes prior to presentation, fall within the category of acquired esotropia and are treated on this basis. If this occurs in the presence of an immature visual system, suppression replaces normal fusion and amblyopia increasingly dominates the clinical picture. The presence of hypermetropia and a history of accommodative strabismus is not uncommon. In such cases the state of fusion and underlying binocular vision may be normal or on the basis of a monofixation syndrome which decompensates.

In adults acute onset of acquired esotropias, particularly in the absence of a family history or significant hypermetropia, requires a neurological examination and neuroimaging. Acquired esotropia may persist after recovery from a sixth nerve palsy whether this be isolated or associated with raised intracranial pressure such as in benign intracranial hypertension, occasionally craniostenosis or sagittal sinus thrombosis seen more commonly in childhood with suppurative middle ear infections.

For acquired esotropia of sudden onset with loss of fusion, neurological examination with neuroimaging, to exclude cerebral neoplasm or other pathology, is essential.

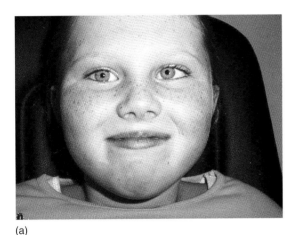

(a)

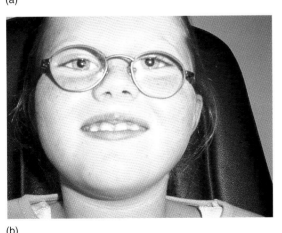

(b)

Figure 4.4 Fully accommodative esotropia in a child. Note full correction of convergent strabismus by hypermetropic spectacles

Fully accommodative

A hypermetropic child who begins to accommodate from the age of 1–3 years may develop an esotropia from overconvergence associated with extra accommodation to correct the hypermetropic error. Such a strabismus is defined to be fully accommodative if the optical correction straightens the eyes completely (Figure 4.4). Although rare, a child with myopia may have straight eyes, but with spectacle correction may present with a manifest esotropia which is clearly accommodative in origin (Figure 4.5).

Partially accommodative

A child's accommodative esotropia reduced by optical correction but not fully eliminated at distance or near is defined as partially accommodative strabismus (Figure 4.6). Such

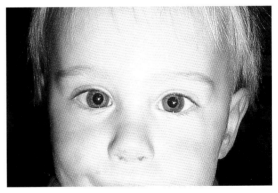

(a)

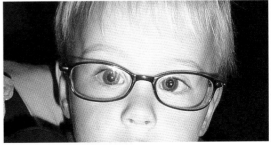

(b)

Figure 4.5 Without glasses (a) the eyes are straight. With glasses (b) the eyes are convergent because of the induced accommodative effort to focus

29

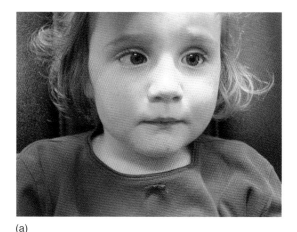

(a)

(b)

Figure 4.6 A partially accommodative esotropia in a child not fully corrected by spectacles

cases are difficult to manage unless promptly diagnosed and managed with occlusion therapy, aimed at eliminating suppression and preventing the onset of amblyopia. Congenital esotropia often with low hypermetropia falls into this group in many cases. Although glasses may not be effective preoperatively, spectacle correction of relatively small degrees of hypermetropia postoperatively can improve alignment sufficiently for monofixation syndrome to evolve.

Esotropia with high AC:A ratio–convergence excess

High AC:A and convergence excess is said to be present when the eyes overconverge for near

viewing of an object in a patient whose refractive error is fully corrected and whose eyes are straight for distance. Although the convergence excess may be present in children of similar age to those with fully accommodative esotropia, it may occur before 6 months and be part of the differential diagnosis of congenital esotropia. It is essential to do a non-dissociating cover test at distance to avoid the wrong diagnosis of constant esotropia.

Such convergence excess esotropias are characterised by accommodation-associated over-convergence, with the esotropia at near often more than 20 dioptres greater than for distance. Patients may be hypermetropic, have a small degree of hypermetropia, or be emmetropic. More rarely, the patient is myopic and the overconvergence only becomes manifest on correction of the myopia and the need to focus on near targets through the prescribed glasses is attended by convergence excess. The convergence excess may be worse if the patient is tense or nervous. Patients with high AC:A ratios who have central bifoveal fusion for distance may not experience diplopia at near when the eyes overconverge because of suppression. Over-convergence associated with accommodation tends to lessen with age and to disappear completely by adolescence, though not invariably.

Management includes prescribing the full hypermetropic correction to be worn. There is no evidence that bifocal glasses improve long term outcome.[11] A number of cases of high AC:A ratio esotropias may require surgery because of breakdown of normal binocular vision at distance.[12] If further cycloplegic refraction reveals no uncorrected hypermetropia, surgery should be deferred to evaluate the full effect of glasses.

Cyclic esotropia (alternate day syndrome)

This is an unusual condition where there are alternating periods of an esotropia (often 30–40 dioptres) on one day followed by perfectly straight eyes on the next day. The strabismus may be of any type but is most commonly esotropia. The periodicity tends to be in cycles of about 24 hours and if untreated, it may become constant within 6 months. Children with this condition are often older, with good fusion. They experience diplopia on the days when the strabismus is present and have binocular single vision when the eyes are straight. Surgery is associated with a high degree of success and indicated if the condition has remained static.

Iatrogenic esotropia

Prolonged occlusion of one eye (for example, following eyelid surgery) may result in sensory deprivation, disruption of binocular vision and occlusion esotropia. Such patients may have never previously had a strabismus but may have had a history of uncorrected hypermetropia or a family history of strabismus. It may also occur in the treatment of anisometropic amblyopia or trauma causing eyelid swelling.[13] This condition is mirrored clinically in some cases of congenital ptosis (Figures 4.7 and 4.8). Awareness and early recognition of this condition are essential. Reduction in the period of occlusion can reverse this condition.

Functional esotropia

It is well known that emotional state may influence the degree of strabismus present in a patient. It can occur following surgical correction where the eyes have been straight. There may be worsening of esotropia with diplopia, even in the presence of fusion.

Esotropia without fusion potential

A significant number of children with congenital esotropia do not achieve peripheral fusion and stable ocular alignment even though treated early in their visual development and left with small residual squints. Since the majority of children with congenital esotropia would have had ocular alignment by age 2 it is difficult to identify this group. In the siblings and family of

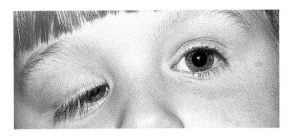

Figure 4.7 A child with convergent strabismus from congenital ptosis disrupting binocular vision

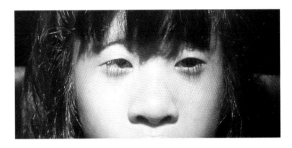

Figure 4.8 A child with concurrent blepharophimosis and right convergent strabismus

some of these children it is our experience that some have defects in their binocular vision and quality of stereopsis and fusion, suggesting there is a defect in the development that remains as the basis for this group. Asymmetrical OKN is present in these cases. The one eye may dominate, with the second eye contributing to the overall visual field. Subsequent consecutive divergence squints may occur.

Esotropia in cerebral palsy

Strabismus and indeed visual abnormalities are common in hydrocephalus and cerebral palsy. Although esotropia is more common, other ocular deviations reflecting a different neurologic basis may be the reason for presentation.

The inclination to correct these cases deserves more attention. Parents often state that with the straightening of eyes the child's general performance improves. It is more likely that the improved appearance of the child results in the child being treated with more consideration by teachers and their peers.

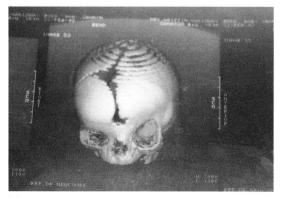

(a)

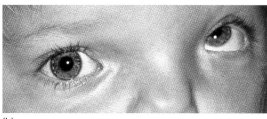

(b)

Figure 4.9 Craniosynostosis is a maldevelopment of the orbit and of individual ocular muscles associated with premature closure of one or both coronal sutures. Note the left coronal synostosis in the polytomogram (a) and the disturbed growth of the left orbit with the upper outer angle pointing to the synostosis. The clinical photo (b) shows the flattening of the left forehead and the upwardly displaced eyebrow, together with evidence of weakness of the left superior oblique muscle which in this case had a lax tendon

Childhood exotropias

Constant childhood exotropia

In most children exotropia is intermittent. An occasional child has a constant exotropia and an inability to align the eyes. This should alert the clinician to associated pathology. Constant exotropia is associated with craniosynostosis syndromes, which constitute a large part of craniofacial syndromes. They are characterised by premature closure of one or more cranial or facial bony sutures, resulting in abnormal growth patterns and altered shape of the skull (Figure 4.9). Multiple suture involvement may result in raised intracranial pressure. Well known

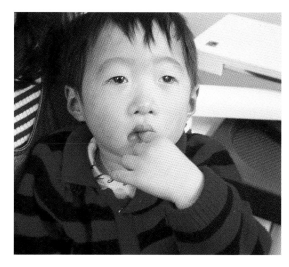

Figure 4.10 A child with suspected perinatal ischaemia with a constant divergent strabismus and global developmental delay with some dysmorphic features, including absence of lacrimal apparatus

syndromes include Apert's and Crouzon's. Patients with these conditions may demonstrate a range of esotropias, although exotropia is more common. A commonly found pattern is a V pattern on upgaze and an esotropia on downgaze. In a number of patients, muscles are abnormal, small, or have abnormal insertions when found at surgery or CT scan. Pathology associated with constant exotropias of this sort may have a number of aetiologies. Mild cases may not be obvious but the clinician should look for them when confronted with a child with a constant exotropia.

A second source of constant exotropia is neurologic damage. Children with perinatal ischaemia may lose their ability to use their eyes together and develop a constant exotropia. Constant exotropia is so uncommon in the first few years of life as to warrant a very careful investigation for craniofacial or neurologic injury (Figure 4.10).

Differential diagnoses of constant exotropias should include the so-called pseudo exotropia caused by dragging of the macula. Pseudo exotropia occurs, for example, in children with temporal dragging of the macula caused by retinopathy of prematurity or inflammatory lesions such as toxocara. As the macula is drawn temporally, the eye must be extorted to align the visual axis. Essentially, the visual angle changes, causing the child to appear exotropic. However, diagnostic tests for strabismus will demonstrate there is no actual misalignment of the visual axis. Recognition of pseudo exotropia is important because any effort to fix this surgically is bound to fail.

Constant exotropia is managed in most cases with a surgical procedure. The surgeon should consider the underlying craniofacial and neurologic status of the child before this is undertaken. In some cases amblyopia requires management. Optical correction of constant exotropia is not nearly as successful as in intermittent exotropias.

Intermittent exotropia

Many children have a transient exotropia in the first weeks of life that can be regarded as a variant of normal development. By contrast intermittent exotropia presents usually before the age of 18 months. It may be first noticed when the child is unwell and the eye drifts out. There may be a family history of strabismus and small degrees of exotropia can often be controlled. Closure of the divergent eye in sunlight is not an uncommon initial presentation. "Squint" for many in the community means closure of one or both eyes. When children are described as having a squint, it is therefore important to clarify if the family notices a deviation of the eye, as opposed to closure of one eye in sunlight. Closure of one eye in sunlight may be part of a normal response to glare. It may in addition be the result of an eye movement disorder, or the result of a disorder of refractive media, pupil, retina, or optic nerve.

A not uncommon feature of intermittent exotropia is the high degree of stereoacuity for near objects. Intermittent exotropia implies a breakdown of normal binocular vision at distance (Figure 4.11). By definition there is a high degree of binocular vision for near objects.

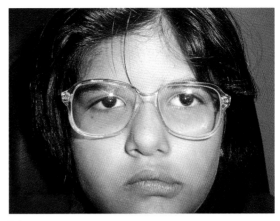

(a)

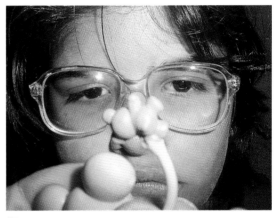

(b)

Figure 4.11 Intermittent exotropia in a child whose binocular vision has broken down for distance and is thus divergent for distance but is binocular for near targets

However, once suppression occurs, the eye deviates out. Since double vision does not occur when the eye becomes divergent, it would appear that suppression in the deviating eye is extensive over the hemiretina. This may involve mechanisms of motor fusion during the development of normal binocular vision. During examination, it is very important to get the patient to fix on a near object of interest, and to demonstrate normal single binocular vision and challenge the binocular vision with prisms (see Chapter 6).

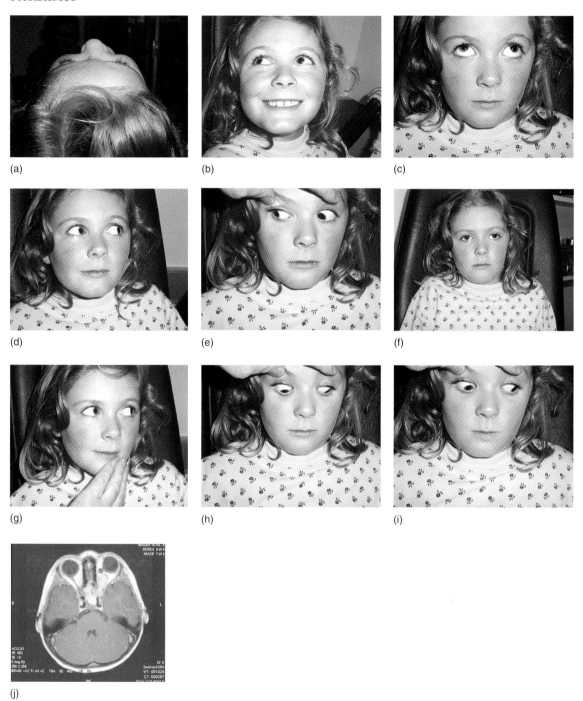

Figure 4.12 Strabismus associated with optic chiasm glioma. The parents of this child noted an intermittent left divergent squint at 18 months. She presented at the age of 5 years with a divergent strabismus, unusual eye movements, left myelinated nerve fibres, mild proptosis (a), and left disc pallor. There were no café au lait spots. (NB Café au lait spots may not be present before the age of 6 months.) Unusual eye movements were demonstrated as shown (b-i). The MRI demonstrated a chiasmal glioma (j). In patients with eye movement disorders in the presence of neurofibromatosis, there is a case for MRI at an early stage

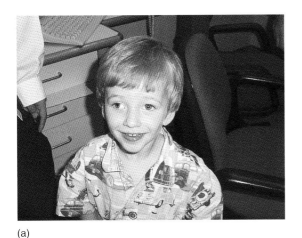

(a)

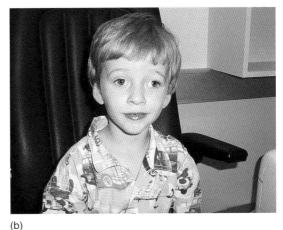

(b)

Figure 4.13 Alternating divergent strabismus. Constant alternating divergent strabismus in a 3 year old child. Note alternation of fixation. Most children have a transient exotropia in the first weeks of life. It is important to exclude any neurological deficits. This child had no binocular vision in the absence of a neurological defect

Though the vast majority of Intermittent exotropias are probably the result of a static underlying cause, it is important to keep in mind any clue alerting the clinician to a possible loss of visual field, frustrating sufficient overlapping to meet the needs of normal binocular vision.

Congenital exotropia that persists is a different matter. A large angle up to 50 prism dioptres may be present with a constant exotropia. Because of the frequency of associated neurological disease, referral to a paediatric neurologist is advised. Differential diagnosis includes developmental defects in the deviating eye and congenital cranial nerve palsies. Local causes of defective vision need to be excluded. A careful developmental history will frequently reveal abnormal milestones if there is underlying neurological disease. In the context of neurological disease, for example neurofibromatosis, the exotropia may signal the presence of a progressive disease (Figure 4.12), frequently affecting the sensory arc of the visual path. Early surgery by the age of 2 years will achieve a more stable alignment for distance, but is often at the cost of a monofixation syndrome. Surgery by the age of 4 or 5 years appears to be associated with a higher risk of intermittent divergence persisting. Surgery for patients under the age of 4 years gives complete cure in about 50% of cases. Lateral incomitance may exist in about 5% of exotropes,[10] and needs to be identified as a failure to recognise it may result in surgical overcorrections. It is also important to note that a child with an alternating divergent fixation present at distance and near may have no underlying neurological defect (Figure 4.13).

Management

The options in management include minus lenses in glasses if the patient is myopic. Deliberate overcorrection with concave lenses aims to induce accommodation to assist control of the deviation, and may have a limited place in management. Surgical correction involves bilateral lateral rectus recessions up to 11 mm from the limbus. Medial rectus resection in patients with a convergence insufficiency type of exophoria also has a limited value. Complications of surgery include underactions in over 25% of cases. Surgical alignment occurs in as many as 80% with good cosmetic prospects, but only 50% have good binocular vision after surgery.

35

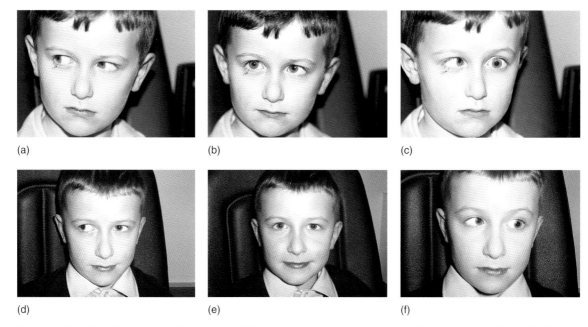

(a)   (b)   (c)

(d)   (e)   (f)

Figure 4.14   Left Duane's syndrome in a child before (a, b, c) and after surgical correction (d, e, f) with the Carlson-Jampolsky procedure. Note in right gaze the narrowing of the left palpebral aperture in left gaze the widening of the left palpebral aperture

Incomitant strabismus

Horizontal movement disorders

Sixth nerve palsy associated with syndromes such as Duane's and Moebius' need to be distinguished from transient neonatal sixth nerve palsies.[14]

Duane retraction syndrome

Duane syndrome is an unusual condition where there is a deficit of horizontal movement associated with a paradoxical innervation of horizontal muscles[15] (Figure 4.14). The deficit of movement may be partial or incomplete.

Huber classification is clinical and still the most widely used today and subdivides Duane retraction syndrome into three subtypes.

Type I is three times as common as type II and III combined and presents with esotropia and marked limitation of abduction with minimally defective adduction. There is retraction of the palpebral fissure in adduction and widening of the fissure in abduction with characteristic paradoxical innervation of the LR on adduction.

Type II shows marked limitation of adduction with exotropia of the affected eye; paradoxical innervation of the lateral rectus occurs in both abduction and adduction. There is retraction and narrowing of the palpebral fissure on attempted adduction.

In type III, there is combined limitation, or both adduction and abduction, and narrowing of the globe and palpebral fissures on attempted adduction. Electromyograph findings show intense innervation of both the lateral and medial rectus whether in primary gaze adduction or abduction.

Most commonly Duane syndrome is an isolated abnormality but may also accompany sensory hearing loss and a constellation of other systemic syndromes.

Additional ocular defects include a tendency towards anisometropia, a slightly increased incidence of optic nerve abnormalities, and the

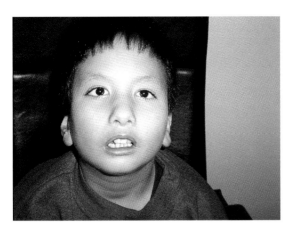

Figure 4.15 Moebius syndrome. The ocular features include cranial sixth and seventh nerve palsies. However, gaze palsies are equally common and may be combined with these palsies. Bimedial rectus recession will produce good ocular alignment but often at the expense of convergence

chance that amblyopia will develop. Duane syndrome is occasionally bilateral, although it has a predilection for the left eye. For further management of Duane syndrome see Chapter 7.

Moebius syndrome

Moebius syndrome consists of congenital disturbance of eye movements and facial diplegia (Figure 4.15). Accompanying features include deformities of the head and face, atrophy of the tongue, endocrine abnormalities and malformations of the chest, including defects of the pectoralis muscles, malformations of the lower limbs and extremities. Ocular features of Moebius syndrome include sixth and seventh cranial nerve palsies with bilateral abduction deficits, accompanied by bilateral facial nerve weakness.

Many display a horizontal gaze palsy with convergence substitution movements rather than a sixth nerve palsy. Moebius syndrome is most likely due to congenital compromise of the abducens nerve, facial nerve and pontine parareticular formation (PPRF). Neurovascular

insult and the possibility of teratogens have been implicated, due to their effect on the developing vasculature of the brain.[16] In some cases, a pendular nystagmus is present. Patients with a congenital absence of horizontal conjugate eye movements may adapt strategies to compensate for this. They substitute head saccades for eye saccades and if the head is immobilised they may use an intact vergence system to move the eyes into abduction and then cross-fixate. In Moebius syndrome it is important to differentiate this from cases where there are sixth and seventh nerve palsies. It is possible that this mechanism is more common in Moebius syndrome than previously supposed and that it may be confused for the more commonly diagnosed combined nerve palsies.

Congenital myotonic dystrophy, congenital horizontal gaze palsy and Duane syndrome can all be confused with this syndrome. Moebius syndrome may be accompanied by a variety of systemic findings as well.

There is an unanswered question as to why aberrant innervation seen in Duane syndrome is so rarely seen as part of Moebius syndrome. What is of interest is how frequently bilateral medial recession corrects the deviation, suggesting that there is residual tone in the lateral rectus, although patients may still be left with defective convergence.

At surgery, children with Moebius syndrome may have extremely tight medial rectus muscles. This may be caused by the fact that they are unopposed by defective lateral rectus muscles and therefore develop constriction and tightness. Large medial rectus recessions are indicated and will usually serve the purpose of straightening the eyes in primary gaze. This contrasts with the unrewarding results of medial rectus recession for complete sixth nerve palsy.

Sixth nerve palsy

Acquired sixth nerve palsies in childhood may be secondary to neurological disease, hydrocephalus, transverse sinus thrombosis,

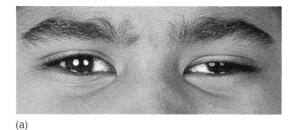

(a)

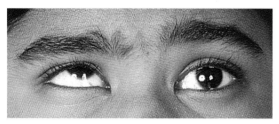

(b)

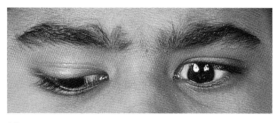

(c)

Figure 4.16　Child (a–c) with left ptosis due to third nerve palsy

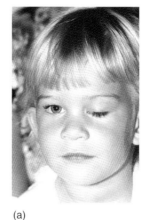

(a)

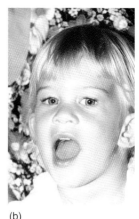

(b)

Figure 4.17　Developmentally determined aberrant innervation resulting in the Marcus Gunn jaw winking syndrome

tumour of nasopharynx, trauma, infections, (Gradenigo syndrome), and vascular malformation.

Benign sixth nerve palsy of childhood can also occur in infancy when associated with febrile illness. It is transitory and recovers within weeks.[17–19] It is important to distinguish benign sixth nerve palsy from pontine glioma if it does not resolve within 6 weeks.

Third nerve palsy

This condition may be congenital. The palsy is usually unilateral but less commonly bilateral. The pupil may be spared and the condition may be associated with aberrant regeneration. Third nerve palsy is associated with ophthalmoplegic migraine in adolescent and early adult life as well

as with posterior cerebral artery aneurysms or vascular malformations. Traumatic causes include uncal herniation in severe head trauma.[20,21,22]

Recovery may be associated with aberrant regeneration and paradoxical movements (Figure 4.16). Another common developmental aberrant regeneration involves the miswiring between motor fifth nerve and eyelid movement from seventh nerve innervations of the orbicularis. It results in the jaw winking phenomenon (Figure 4.17).

Superior oblique paresis

Superior oblique paresis is relatively common in childhood (Figure 4.18). The weakness may be a true fourth nerve palsy but a significant number are due to developmental anomalies of the superior oblique muscle, particularly its tendon. The child usually presents later in infancy with a compensatory torticollis. There may be inferior oblique overaction and a positive Bielschowsky head tilt test (Figure 4.19). Approximately one quarter of superior oblique palsies are congenital. Some cases of apparent congenital fourth nerve palsy have been

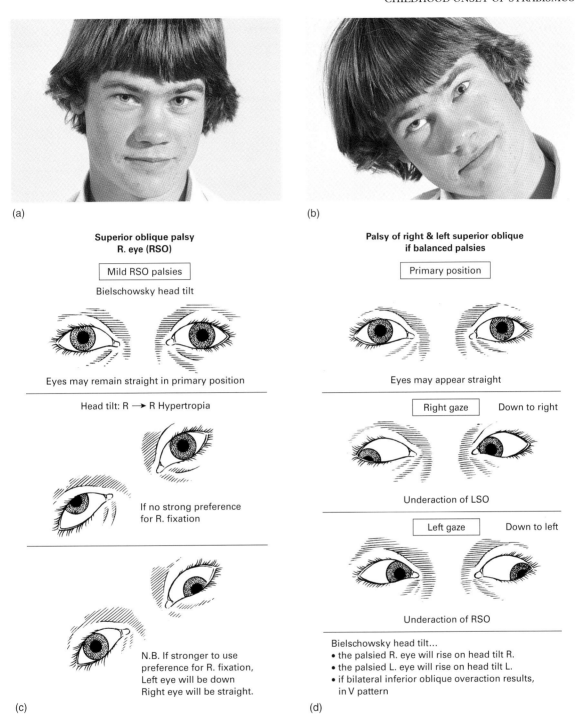

(a)

(b)

**Superior oblique palsy
R. eye (RSO)**

Mild RSO palsies

Bielschowsky head tilt

Eyes may remain straight in primary position

Head tilt: R → R Hypertropia

If no strong preference
for R. fixation

N.B. If stronger to use
preference for R. fixation,
Left eye will be down
Right eye will be straight.

(c)

**Palsy of right & left superior oblique
if balanced palsies**

Primary position

Eyes may appear straight

Right gaze   Down to right

Underaction of LSO

Left gaze   Down to left

Underaction of RSO

Bielschowsky head tilt...
• the palsied R. eye will rise on head tilt R.
• the palsied L. eye will rise on head tilt L.
• if bilateral inferior oblique overaction results,
 in V pattern

(d)

Figure 4.18 Superior oblique paresis. (a) Note the AHP with face turn left and head tilt left to maintain binocular single vision. (b) With head tilt to right (Bielschowsky head tilt test) the underacting right superior oblique muscle is unable to control the muscle imbalance. The right eye elevates and binocular single vision is broken down. Diagram (c) further illustrates unilateral weakness of the right superior oblique muscle. Diagram (d) demonstrates the findings anticipated in bilateral superior oblique weakness

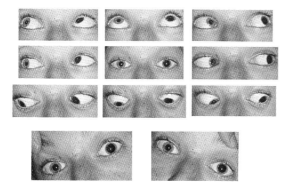

Figure 4.19 Left traumatic fourth nerve palsy demonstrating weakness of left superior oblique muscle. Note left hypertropia, worse in right gaze and left head tilt (Bielschowsky head tilt test). Note also traumatic left mydriasis

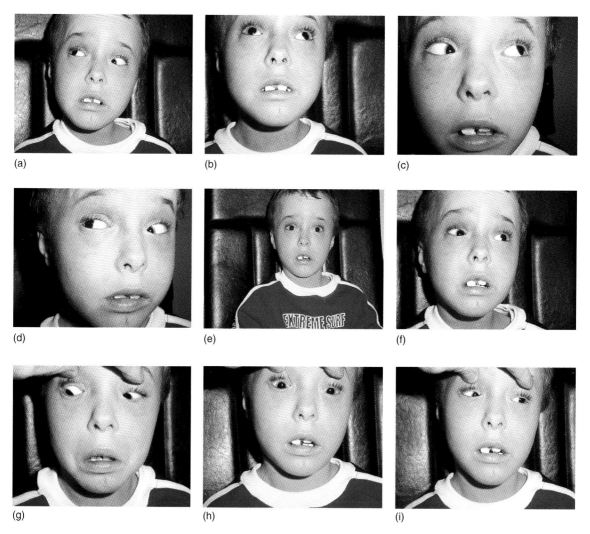

(a)　(b)　(c)

(d)　(e)　(f)

(g)　(h)　(i)

Figure 4.20 Child with bilateral Brown's syndrome. Note in right and left gaze the adducting eye turns down and is unable to elevate due to tightness of the superior oblique tendon. Note also in moving from depression to elevation in the mid-line the pattern of movement is a V due to the eye pivoting about the anchored attachment of the superior oblique. The clinician should suspect Brown's syndrome when there is a V pattern of movement in the presence of apparent underacting inferior obliques

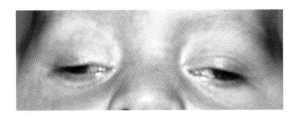

Figure 4.21 Congenital fibrosis syndrome is characterised by a bilateral ptosis, divergent squint, eyes in depression, and inability to elevate them. There is markedly restricted vertical movement and attempts to depress the eyes result in further divergence

demonstrated to have laxity of the superior oblique tendon. Anomalies of the reflected tendon of superior oblique include:

- a redundant tendon

- a misdirected tendon inserting on the nasal border of superior rectus

- an attenuated tendon inserting to the under-surface of Tenon's capsule, or

- an absent tendon.

Absence of superior oblique is occasionally associated with craniofacial synostosis.[23–25]

Vertical movement disorders of early infancy

Isolated inferior oblique palsy

This is an extremely rare form of uniocular muscle paresis. It is usually congenital, rarely traumatic and is diagnosed with the findings of hypertropia with a head tilt toward the side of the hypertropic eye. Convergence in upgaze (A pattern) contrasts with the exotropia on upgaze (V pattern) seen in Brown's syndrome (Figure 4.20, see also chapter 7, p78) and helps in the differential diagnosis of inability to elevate the eye in adduction.

Transient skew deviation

Described in neonates, this condition is rare and transient. It has been described as a transient palsy in obstetric trauma in otherwise healthy neonates. By contrast, persistent skew deviation of the eyes, although rare, is found in association with brainstem disease. Skew deviation has to be distinguished from primary inferior oblique over action (see chapter 4, p26). Skew deviation with brainstem disease can present as the classical "setting sun" sign, with tonic looking down of the eyes and lid retraction most commonly seen with hydrocephalus or kernicterus.

Benign paroxysmal tonic upgaze of childhood

This recently described syndrome in contrast to the "setting sun" sign is an apparently benign oculomotor disorder with onset in early life.[26] Characteristic features include episodes of sustained upgaze, with downbeating saccades in attempted downgaze which are difficult to sustain below the primary position. There are apparently normal horizontal movements. Sleep gives relief. The cases we have seen have otherwise normal neurological findings apart from ataxia. We noted the absence of deterioration during observation over 15 years, with improvement of symptoms in some patients.

Congenital fibrosis syndrome

This is an autosomal dominant condition associated with abnormal neuronal migration and fixed hypodeviation of both eyes (Figures 4.21 and 4.22). Head tilt with chin elevation, and a spastic convergence on attempted lateral or upgaze are also associated features.

Recent studies of these cases in our department and Westmead Children's Hospital have demonstrated abnormalities of the lateral ventricle and basal nuclei suggesting that the fibrosis of ocular muscles is due to static pathology associated with a developmental central nervous system disorder. These findings

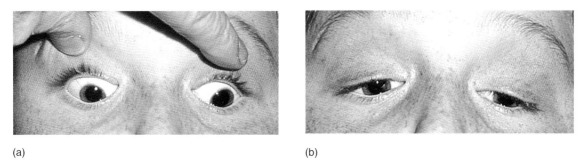

(a)   (b)

Figure 4.22   Young boy with congenital fibrosis syndrome, characterised by bilateral ptosis, divergent strabismus, markedly restricted vertical movement and increased divergence on attempts to depress or elevate the eyes

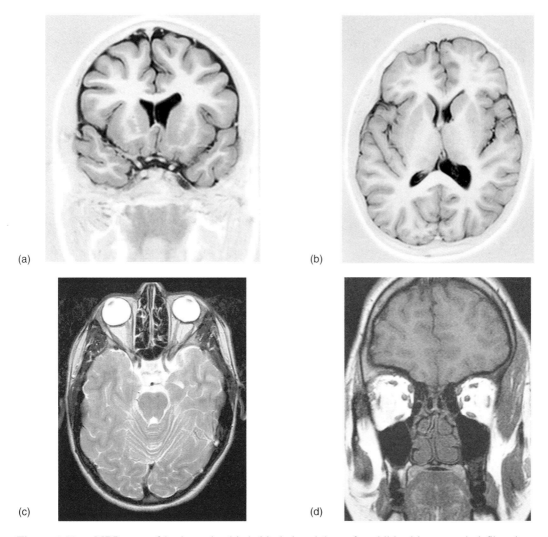

(a)   (b)

(c)   (d)

Figure 4.23   MRI scan of brain and orbit behind the globes of a child with congenital fibrosis syndrome, showing fusion of the left caudate nucleus head and underlying lentiform nucleus (a), atrophy of the left caudate body and tail with enlargement of the ipsilateral ventricle (b). There is also hypoplasia of medial and superior recti and some fibrosis of the lateral recti (c, d)

add weight to the theme of this book that, in cases of strabismus, the underlying cause may be lesions (sensory or motor) resulting in disturbed binocular movement. The pathology may be static but, more importantly, it may be slowly progressive, for example gliomas of the visual path, with no other clinical manifestations than skin lesions that provide a clue to the diagnosis.

In severe cases, there is bilateral complete ptosis, divergent strabismus and no elevation or depression of the eyes. In such cases, elevation of the lids may aggravate exposure keratitis and ocular muscle surgery is unrewarding. These full-blown cases are associated with structural change as reported by Flaherty and Gillies (Figure 4.23).

We have also observed sporadic cases without widespread cortical dysplasia or other clinically significant features. The possibility that sporadic cases represent a distinct group or form part of a spectrum requires further study.

Opsoclonus

Opsoclonus is a rapid to and fro movement of the eyes which has been described in children with encephalitis and hydrocephalus. Opsoclonus may present in infants with occult neuroblastoma that demands neurological evaluation.

Internuclear ophthalmoplegia

Internuclear ophthalmoplegia is occasionally seen in premature infants, possibly related to immaturity of the medial longitudinal fasciculus.

Neonatal myasthenia gravis

Clinical manifestations of paediatric disorders of the neuromuscular junction depend on the mechanism and severity of the defect and age of patient. Ptosis, strabismus, and internuclear ophthalmoplegia have all been observed.

This disorder is seen in 10–15% of infants born to mothers with autoimmune myasthenia gravis. The risk is greater if there are affected siblings. Patients with neonatal myasthenia gravis are symptomatic at birth with facial weakness, dysphagia, weak suck and respiratory insufficiency.

Diagnostic tests for neonatal myasthenia include antibodies to acetylcholine receptors and electrodiagnostic findings similar to adults, including descending repetitive stimulation amplitudes with a normal compound muscle action potential.

Congenital myasthenia occurs in infants born to non-myasthenic mothers. This ophthalmoplegia is not usually present in the neonatal period. External ophthalmoplegia may be a result of food-borne or wound botulinum.

Other eye movement disorders – associations with strabismus

There are a number of eye movement disorders that present to clinicians with an interest in strabismus. They are important because they may be associated with strabismus but in most cases they raise questions as to underlying aetiology and the possibility of neurologic disease.

Congenital nystagmus

Congenital nystagmus is not usually manifested until the early months of life. Nystagmus has been divided according to whether the underlying cause is thought to be sensory or motor. However, the characteristics of the particular movement disorder in the nystagmus do not in themselves provide a distinction between the two.

In some cases where the underlying basis is sensory there may be an associated head posture. The importance of this is that there may be delay in diagnosis of a cerebral tumour such as optic nerve glioma or craniopharyngioma affecting the chiasm if the nystagmus is misdiagnosed as motor nystagmus.[27] We found half the infants under 5 years with optic chiasmal

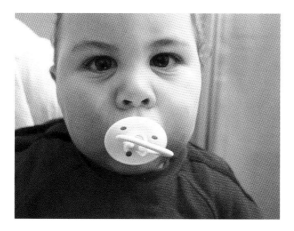

Figure 4.24 Left convergent strabismus in a child with oculomotor apraxia, noted to have head thrusting movements at 6 months (MRI shown in Fig 4.25)

gliomas had nystagmus.[28] Sensory causes are more commonly static but the diagnosis can depend on the recognition of subtle signs. A good rule is to assume the cause is sensory until proved otherwise.

Sensory causes difficult to diagnose include macular coloboma, toxoplasmosis and many conditions that have an hereditary basis. Foveal hypoplasia may be associated with albinism or with complete aniridia. Oculocutaneous albinism is usually obvious and is recessive in its inheritance. Ocular albinism, less obvious clinically, is usually X-linked, although 10% are recessive.[29] Iris transillumination should be looked for, and also in the mother. Other conditions include Leber retinal dystrophy, often suspected on its other association with high hypermetropia. This condition also requires genetic counselling as do congenital night blindness and rod partial monochromatism.

Motor nystagmus is most often associated with a null point for the nystagmus and abnormal head posture. This may be in any particular direction of gaze for the particular case, usually in a conjugate field of gaze. By contrast, in cases of Ciancia syndrome the null point in each eye will be in a position of convergence.

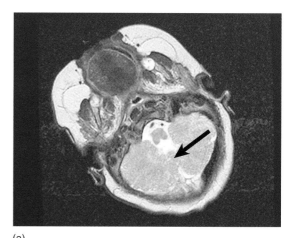

(a)

(b)

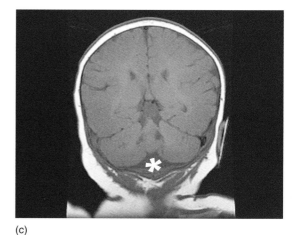

(c)

Figure 4.25 MRI scan of child with oculomotor apraxia showing hypoplasia of the cerebellar vermis (arrow) (a) and enlarged cisterna magna (asterisk) (b, c)

Spasmus nutans

This condition is characterised by nodding spasms which are self-limiting. It was originally regarded as a benign condition characterised by asymmetric acquired pendular nystagmus, head nodding and head tilt. There is a typical age of onset with nystagmus preceding head nodding at between 4–12 months. What is important is that there are no reliable diagnostic clues to differentiate spasmus nutans from acquired pendular nystagmus and intracranial tumours, including chiasmal gliomas.

Congenital retraction nystagmus

Attempts to look up are associated with eyeball retraction. The movement is thought to be due to opposed saccades. Clinically there may be associated dorsal midbrain lesions which may be intrinsic, for example Parinaud syndrome, or extrinsic, for example hydrocephalus.

Ocular motor apraxia

Harris introduced the term saccade initiation failure (SIF). Strabismus is common (see Figure 4.24). SIF is intermittent, often more noticeable when the child is stressed or tired. In congenital SIF, the saccades when they occur have normal speeds. Head thrusting (see glossary for definition) may not develop until 2–3 months. Shifting gaze with the head may also compensate for gaze palsy, hemianopia, slow saccades or even poor eccentric gaze holding. Older children facilitate the triggering of saccades by blinking synkinetically. Apart from agenesis of the corpus callosum most structural abnormalities associated with SIF occur in the posterior fossa, around the fourth ventricle and vermis (Figure 4.25). MRI is preferred. There is no treatment for SIF. Visual outcome is good, although delayed speech and poor reading as well as clumsiness and educational problems may be apparent later in development.

Periodic alternating nystagmus

Periodic alternating nystagmus is seen as a congenital nystagmus. It is characterised by repeated cycles of nystagmus alternating in the direction of beating punctuated by a pause in the movement disorder. It is important to exclude posterior fossa neurologic disease and to be aware of the association with Arnold–Chiari malformation, congenital hydrocephalus, and myelomeningocele.

References

1. Calcutt C. The natural history of infantile esotropia. A study of the untreated condition in the visual adult. *Advances in Amblyopia and Strabismus*. Transactions of the VIIth International Orthoptic Congress, Nurnberg, 1991.
2. Phillips CI. Anisometropic amblyopia, axial length in strabismus and some observations on spectacle correction. *Br Orthopt J* 1966;**23**:57–61.
3. Hiles DA, Watson BA, Biglan AW. Characteristics of infantile esotropia following early bimedial rectus recession. *Arch Ophthalmol* 1980;**98**:697–703.
4. Calcutt C, Murray AD. Untreated essential infantile esotropia: factors affecting the development of amblyopia. *Eye* 1998;**12**:167–72.
5. Ing MR. The timing of surgical alignment for congenital (infantile) esotropia. *J Pediatr Ophthalmol Strabismus* 1999;**36**:61–8;85–6.
6. Murray A. *Natural History of Untreated Strabismus*. Argentina, 2001.
7. Helveston EM. Dissociated vertical deviation: a clinical and laboratory study. *Trans Am Ophthalmol Soc* 1981;**78**:734.
8. Lang J. Der Kongenitale oder Fruhkindliche Strabismus. *Ophthalmologica* 1967;**154**:201.
9. Ciancia AO. On infantile esotropia with nystagmus in abduction. *J Pediatr Ophthalmol Strabismus* 1995;**32**:280–8.
10. Kushner BJ. Ocular causes of abnormal head postures. *Ophthalmology* 1979;**86**:2115–25.
11. Pratt-Johnson JA, Tillson G. The management of esotropia with high AC/A ratio (convergence excess). *J Pediatr Ophthalmol Strabismus* 1985;**22**:238–42.
12. Ludwig IH, Parks MM, Getson PR, Kammerman LA. Rate of deterioration in accommodative esotropia correlated to the AC/A relationship. *J Pediatr Ophthalmol Strabismus* 1988;**25**:8–12.
13. von Noorden GK, ed. *Binocular Vision and Ocular Motility*. St Louis: Mosby, 1990.
14. Reisner SH, Perlman M, Ben-Tovim N, Dubrawski C. Transient lateral rectus muscle paresis in the newborn infant. *J Pediatr* 1971;**78**:461–5.
15. Hotchkiss MG, Miller NR, Clark AW, Green WR. Bilateral Duane's retraction syndrome. A clinical-pathologic case report. *Arch Ophthalmol* 1980;**98**:870–4.
16. Lipson AH, Webster WS, Brown-Woodman PD, Osborn RA. Moebius syndrome: animal model–human correlations and evidence for a brainstem vascular etiology. *Teratology* 1989;**40**:339–50.
17. Robertson DM, Hines JD, Rucker CW. Acquired sixth-nerve paresis in children. *Arch Ophthalmol* 1970;**83**:574–9.

18. Bixenman WW, von Noorden GK. Benign recurrent VI nerve palsy in childhood. *J Pediatr Ophthalmol Strabismus* 1981;**18**:29–34.
19. Harley RD. Paralytic strabismus in children. Etiologic incidence and management of the third, fourth, and sixth nerve palsies. *Ophthalmology* 1980;**87**:24–43.
20. Balkan R, Hoyt CS. Associated neurologic abnormalities in congenital third nerve palsies. *Am J Ophthalmol* 1984;**97**:315–9.
21. Good WV, Barkovich AJ, Nickel BL, Hoyt CS. Bilateral congenital oculomotor nerve palsy in a child with brain anomalies. *Am J Ophthalmol* 1991;**111**:555–8.
22. Schumacher-Feero LA, Yoo KW, Solari FM, Biglan AW. Third cranial nerve palsy in children. *Am J Ophthalmol* 1999;**128**:216–21.
23. Ellis FD, Helveston EM. Superior oblique palsy: diagnosis and classification. *Int Ophthalmol Clin* 1976;**16**:127–35.
24. Plager DA. Traction testing in superior oblique palsy. *J Pediatr Ophthalmol Strabismus* 1990;**27**:136–40.
25. Plager DA. Tendon laxity in superior oblique palsy. *Ophthalmology* 1992;**99**:1032–8.
26. Ouvrier RA, Billson FA. Benign paroxysmal tonic upgaze of childhood. *J Child Neurol* 1988;**3**:177–80.
27. Chutorian AM, Schwartz JF. Optic gliomas in children. *Neurology* 1964;**14**:83.
28. Billson FA. Tumours of the eye and orbit. In: Jones PC, Campbell PE, eds. *Tumours of Infancy and Childhood*. Oxford: Blackwell Scientific, 1976.
29. Good WV, Jan JE, DeSa L, Barkovich AJ, Groenveld M, Hoyt CS. Cortical visual impairment in children. *Surv Ophthalmol* 1994;**38**:351–64.

5 Adult strabismus

Introduction

The ocular movement disorders of the adult patient attending the ophthalmologist can be thought of as belonging to two distinct groups: those in which the strabismus dates from early childhood (manifest or compensated for, for example by abnormal head posture) and a group that has its onset and aetiology in adult life.

There are significant motor and sensory differences between adult and childhood onset strabismus. The characteristics of adult onset strabismus are mechanical adaptive changes whereas those in childhood occur in the context of the plasticity of a developing brain and visual system. In adults amblyopia does not occur. Problems of abnormal AC:A ratios are rare and usually residua from childhood.

Strabismus of childhood origin in the adult

Untreated childhood strabismus (for example, intermittent exotropia, congenital esotropia) that presents in the adult may be compensated for by abnormal head posture. Patients frequently have equal vision, freely alternating eyes and less risk of amblyopia.

Patients with strabismus with its origin in childhood are of interest, particularly if they have been untreated. Adult patients with untreated strabismus since childhood provide information about the natural history of untreated strabismus from childhood. This contrasts with long-term outcomes from early surgery in childhood.

Untreated intermittent exotropia, although cosmetically obvious, tends to retain excellent binocular vision for near. Early surgical correction of exotropia in children less than 4 years provides more stable ocular alignment, but is accompanied by a higher incidence of monofixation syndrome.

When surgery is performed for intermittent exotropia after the age of 4–5 years, the risk of the monofixation syndrome becomes less as does the ability to achieve a stable ocular alignment in the distance.

Congenital esotropia forms an interesting contrast. The untreated cases show a higher persistence of alternating fixation and only a limited degree of amblyopia.[1-3] Again, this is in contrast to the findings of paediatric strabismus surgeons who strive to align the eyes before the age of 2 years. They then find that the price of a stable ocular alignment is a monofixation syndrome and increased risk of amblyopia. Many adult patients, particularly those without fusion, have cosmetically noticeable strabismus. These cases may include cases surgically aligned in childhood subsequently developing consecutive exotropia, which requires treatment.

The development of consecutive exotropia may present to the ophthalmologist with diplopia because when moving to exotropia, the visual axis for each eye falls outside the retinal suppression area.

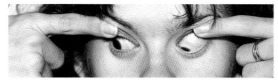

(a)

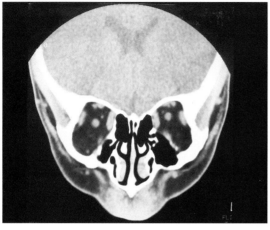

(b)

Figure 5.1 (a) Young woman with congenital absence of both inferior rectus muscles. Note underacting right inferior rectus and features of Rieger's syndrome. (b) MRI of the patient confirming absence of the muscle

Other developmental anomalies, for example congenital absence of rectus muscles, may also continue to cause strabismus in adult life. These syndromes may be familial conditions (Figure 5.1).

Adult onset of strabismus

Sudden onset of strabismus in adults with breakdown of normal binocular vision in a mature visual system results in diplopia. Adaptations include suppression or adoption of abnormal head posture. Occasionally decompensation into manifest strabismus in adults occurs when the basic deviation has been present since early life. These presentations are usually based on loss of motor control. Sensory adaptations are not suddenly changed with the loss of motor control. The exception is the occasional spontaneous loss of suppression leading to double vision that develops following either trauma or, rarely, emotional trauma. For example, if an adult patient with long-standing esotropia develops diplopia and cannot fuse, the possibility of intracranial pathology including tumour or vascular lesion as an underlying cause of central fusion loss needs to be considered.

In contrast to childhood strabismus, the basic deviation of adult strabismus is more stable and more likely determined by mechanical factors or extraocular motor abnormality.

History

It is important to establish the background history of the strabismus in adults including a careful history of childhood onset of strabismus and its management. Photographs in childhood are often valuable in that they may reveal an abnormal head posture or evidence that becomes important in the evaluation of the adult.

Examination

Other important points in assessment of the adult with strabismus include refraction and detailed measurements of the squint in all directions of gaze with and without full optical correction. Deviation should also be measured at near fixation, with and without full optical correction. Spectacles make a difference to the deviation and it is important to discuss with the patient that they may still be necessary even though surgery improves the ocular posture.

Diplopia

Diplopia is uncommon in early childhood because of the plasticity of the brain and the ability of the child to suppress. A condition that may be seen in childhood is that of physiologic diplopia. Simple demonstration to the patient may be helpful to explain the cause of diplopia.

Case example

An adult patient presents with double vision and divergent eyes. History may reveal the patient had a convergent squint during visual immaturity. Subsequent divergence following convergence of the eyes when the visual system is mature implies that as an adult, the position of the optic axis has taken the eye out of the suppression area present when convergent. A helpful confirmatory test is to overcorrect the deviation with prisms and see if this eliminates the diplopia.

The diplopia may occur even if the patient is amblyopic. Surgical treatment involves adjustable suture surgery to realign the eye so that there is suppression of the diplopia. In our experience, suppression can occur but may take months or even 1–2 years to occur. Patients are encouraged to use one eye, and reassured that amblyopia is a childhood condition not an adult one. Patients should be encouraged to use the dominant eye, particularly for distance, and to ignore the second image to stimulate suppression. The patient may prefer the non-dominant eye for near tasks and reading.

Loss of fusion with head trauma or cerebral (brainstem) lesion

Diplopia after severe head trauma requires the exclusion of bilateral superior oblique palsy. These patients may have little evidence of palsy except esotropia in downgaze; the bilateral excyclotorsion can be missed unless carefully looked for. The excyclotorsion can be demonstrated with the Maddox Rod test. It can also be confirmed by careful fundus examination and recorded by fundus photography showing in the rotated retina the macula below its normal position. The mature visual system in the adult is unable to develop suppression in a short period of time. Treatment consists of the surgical technique of Harada–Ito, tightening the anterior fibres of the superior oblique muscle.

Severe head trauma may also cause central fusion disruption, as can a cerebral tumour.[4,5] The sudden onset of palsies of more than one oculomotor nerve (third, fourth, sixth) may create diplopia especially if the patient looks into the direction of the weakened muscle(s). In these adult patients with a mature visual system, diplopia occurs in the context of one image falling on the macula in one eye and the second image falling on an extrafoveal area of the retina of the other eye, resulting in diplopia.

Confusion

This results when there is recent onset of strabismus in adults and each fovea sees a different object that cannot be fused. Retinal rivalry ensues and later the eye looking at the object (the dominant eye) may prevail and the confusing image from the other eye be suppressed.

Significance of Hering's Law

Hering's Law of equal innervation of agonist pairs indicates that paired muscles in either eye receive equal stimulus for movement. If one muscle is paretic fixing with the paretic eye in preference to the non-paretic eye, this will cause a greater deviation of the other eye.

The Parks 3-step test

This test can be helpful in identifying paretic vertical muscle in a strabismus by a process of elimination. Red and green filter glasses are worn to break fusion.

- Step 1. Which eye is higher (hypertropic)?
- Step 2. Is the hypertropia worse in left or right gaze?
- Step 3. Is the hypertropia worse in left or right tilt? (Bielschowsky head tilt test)[6]

There is a simple way of determining the suspect muscle using a modification of the 3–step test.

Step 1: If the right eye is higher then it is a weakness of depressors of the right eye or elevators of the left eye.

Step 2A: If the deviation on tilt is worse on the right side, it is an oblique dysfunction.

Step 2B: If the deviation is worse on left gaze, it is the right superior oblique; and if worse on right gaze, then it is the right inferior oblique.

Step 3A: If deviation on tilt is worse on the left side, then it is a rectus dysfunction

Step 3B: Deviation that is worse on left gaze is the right inferior rectus, and if worse on right gaze, it is the left superior rectus.

Investigation of paretic strabismus

Investigation and measurement of horizontal muscle function is readily obtained, whereas vertical muscle dysfunction may require further clinical tests.

Head tilt

In the presence of paretic strabismus, head tilt is presumed to obtain fusion and to avoid diplopia. Simple tests to demonstrate fusion without demonstrating head tilt should be carried out. The head is then tilted to the opposite side to see if fusion is lost and diplopia evoked. If there is vertical muscle paresis, measurement with the paretic muscle will produce larger deviation of the other eye (Hering's Law). In adults, the patient will normally fix with the normal eye, unless the paretic eye has the better vision. By contrast, in developmentally determined strabismus with binocular vision, the abnormal head posture is not uncommon as a consequence of fixing with the eye with restricted movement in the early years.

Vertical muscle imbalance can be measured with the Parks 3-step test. The use of coloured spectacles with the red glass in front of the right eye and green glass in front of the left eye, then asking the patient to fix a light at 6 m means that the coloured glass dissociates the eyes and makes it easier to make measurements.

Forced duction test

The forced duction test is useful in differentiating defective movement due to mechanical restriction of the muscle or muscle paresis. In children, it should be carried out under general anaesthetic at the commencement of surgery. In adults, forced duction tests can be performed in the clinic using topical anaesthesia. The restriction in oblique muscles will be made more evident by pushing the eye back into the orbit, and in recti muscles by pulling forwards.[7] For example, if there is a lateral rectus palsy, grasping the eye in the adducted position and asking the patient to straighten the eye allows the examiner to make some assessment of residual muscle action.

Saccadic velocities

The patient is asked to change fixation between two fixation targets 20–30° apart. The eye with a weak muscle usually shows a slow saccade in the direction of action of the weak muscle, compared with the normal side.

Restrictive causes of adult strabismus

Thyroid eye disease

In thyroid eye disease, the extraocular muscles may be involved in an infiltrative process and can increase their volume by up to six times. The most frequently involved muscles are medial recti and inferior recti. There is an inflammatory infiltrative disorder of the muscle, resulting in fibrosis and restriction of eye movement. One or both eyes may be involved and a range of restrictive muscle disorders may result. It is important to consider thyroid eye disease in any patient presenting with vertical diplopia. There is a variable association between the time of onset of the thyroid eye disease and the other clinical manifestations, for example Graves disease. In a third of cases, the disease may precede thyrotoxicosis, a third may be concurrent with, and a third may occur years after the disease is quiescent. Patients may complain that the normal eye with unrestricted movement may be riding too high or tending to overshoot (Hering's Law). CT and MRI may reveal characteristic thickening of the posterior half of the muscle with normal sized muscle tendons.[8] Principles of management include ensuring the patient is euthyroid, to minimise surgical risks, and waiting for the muscle balance to be stable for at least 6 months before operating. Prisms may help to control the ocular deviation and reduce compensatory head posture. Adjustable "hang back" sutures are preferred when the condition is stable (see Chapter 7). Caution in recession of inferior rectus must be exercised.

Blowout fractures

Classically occurring as a result of blunt injury, such as a fist, elbow or cricket ball, blowout fractures usually involve the floor and/or the medial wall of the orbit, and the fracture may include trapping of the inferior rectus, inferior oblique or their fasciae. Patients should be observed for a few weeks to see if the restrictive strabismus resolves as the oedema subsides. Diagnosis is made clinically from diplopia with anaesthesia over the infraorbital nerve and enophthalmos. Entrapment of the extraocular muscle can be verified with a positive forced duction test and evidence of prolapsed orbital contents into the maxillary sinus from CT and MRI scans. In most patients, functional recovery occurs without surgery. Indications for surgery include persistent diplopia in the primary position, diplopia in the reading position, and enophthalmos. Surgical treatment involves freeing of the muscle, followed by the insertion of a silicone sheet to cover the fracture separating the contents of the orbit from the adjacent sinus. The decision to operate will often be determined by the forced duction test. Blowout fracture may be mimicked by haemorrhage into an inferior rectus muscle and may resolve spontaneously.

Trochlear injury

Injury to the trochlea may mimic Brown syndrome. In some cases the patient displays a "band phenomenon", where they may have a band of normal binocular single vision that includes the primary position. Above and below this band of normal binocular vision they will have diplopia. In such cases, they may be able to drive and read in comfort. More extreme cases may have little or no evidence of normal binocular vision. In this instance, about a 50% success rate can be achieved with surgery similar to that entertained for Brown syndrome. Surgical treatment of restrictive oblique function in adults more often results in a symptomatic unhappy patient than in childhood.

Restriction of extraocular muscles following retinal detachment surgery

This may occur if the encircling band and the sutures fixing it to the globe interfere with extraocular muscle action; for example, the superior oblique, which is not uncommonly involved.

Muscular causes of adult strabismus

Myasthenia gravis

Myasthenia gravis is a not uncommon autoimmune disorder characterised by destruction of acetylcholine receptors on the neuromuscular endplate of skeletal muscles. Myasthenia gravis may also occur in patients with thyroid eye disease and may occur at any age, including infants, but most often in the third and fourth decades. It should be considered in all patients with thyroid eye disease who present with diplopia, particularly if they are exotropic. The condition may mimic any isolated ocular motor palsy or internuclear ophthalmoplegia. The clinician should be alerted particularly if there is an intermittent variability of muscle tone. Ocular involvement is present in 90% of cases and is the presenting feature in over half the cases. Ocular myasthenia usually becomes generalised, within 2 years of onset, but remains restricted to the ocular muscles in about 30% of patients. By generalised is meant beyond the ocular muscles. However, it needs to be recognised that this extension beyond the ocular muscles may extend only to surrounding muscles of the face and not involve the trunk. The diagnosis may involve several tests (see Box 5.1).

Box 5.1 Tests for myasthenia gravis

- Muscle fatigue test – patient looks up for 30 s to demonstrate worsening of ptosis.
- Dark room test – if ptosis resolves, diagnosis confirmed.
- Cogan's twitch sign of overshoot and twitch with straight gaze after downgaze for several minutes is diagnostic.
- Tensilon test – inject 0·2 cc edrophonium chloride. If improvement occurs, this confirms a diagnosis of myasthenia. If no response, inject further until a total of 0·8 cc has been administered. Objective improvement in the muscles being observed confirms a diagnosis of myasthenia. Intravenous atropine should be kept available for adverse response such as abdominal pain and gastrointestinal disturbance. Neostigmine in children pretreated with atropine allows more time for assessment.
- Antibodies to acetylcholine receptors are present in patients with generalised myasthenia and in most patients with ocular myasthenia.
- CT or MRI of the mediastinum should be performed to exclude thymoma, which is more common in children, but may be present in 20–30% of adults, particularly males.

Myositis

Idiopathic orbital myositis may extend to involve a posterior scleritis or anteriorly to involve the lacrimal gland. It is usually painful to pressure and during attempts to move the eye in the direction of the muscle's action, unlike thyroid eye disease. It is unilateral, although it may be bilateral in 25% of cases (more frequently in women). Distinguishing features of myositis on CT and MRI include involvement of both muscle and tendon, in contrast to thyroid eye disease, where the muscle belly is predominantly involved.

Neurological causes of adult strabismus

Third nerve palsy

Disorders of the third nerve can occur anywhere from the midbrain to the orbit at various levels. Its relationship to the tentorial edge as it crosses the subarachnoid space makes it vulnerable to damage from raised intracranial pressure, causing uncal herniation, and also from hydrocephalus and trauma. Palsy of the superior division of the third nerve involves ptosis, an inability to elevate the eye with involvement of the levator muscle and the superior rectus. With injury to the inferior division of the third nerve, there is inability to adduct the eye or to look inferiorly and the pupil can be involved. Pupillomotor fibres run on the superior aspect of the third nerve and ultimately reach the parasympathetic supply to the eye through the inferior division and its branch to the inferior oblique muscle. Aberrant regeneration occurs in the third nerve particularly after a compressive lesion, such as an aneurysm of posterior cerebral or intracranial portion of internal carotid artery or pituitary tumour or following trauma. Third nerve palsy of sudden onset with pupil involvement requires an MRI. If aneurysm is suspected, neurological consultation and angiography is important. Presentation can occur with intermittent vertical diplopia and pupil dilatation as the only sign. If the pupil remains spared, MRI can be deferred, such as in older patients with microvascular disease, particularly in the presence of diabetes mellitus. Compressive lesions may be the cause of a third nerve palsy with pupil sparing. In older patients (60–70 years) who present with cranial nerve palsies, consideration should also be given to the diagnosis of temporal arteritis.

Fourth nerve palsy

The fourth nerve is the longest and most commonly injured cranial nerve. Usually a V pattern of movement due to associated overaction of the inferior oblique muscles occurs. Abnormal head posture with contralateral head tilt, contralateral turn and chin depression is often found. Congenital fourth cranial nerve palsies not uncommonly become symptomatic in adult life. This is due to the increasing muscle imbalance exceeding reserves of fusion. Such patients will have cyclofusional reserve exceeding that anticipated in adult onset fourth nerve palsy. This, together with old photographs showing an abnormal head posture, is diagnostic. Trauma, atherosclerotic microvascular disease and diabetes are the common causes in adult patients. Aetiology of fourth nerve palsies should be considered at a number of different levels.

Sixth nerve palsy

A sixth nerve palsy may affect the nerve anywhere from the pons to its innervation of the lateral rectus. It is important to realise that sixth nerve palsy may occur as a non-localising sign of raised intracranial pressure. Microvascular disease from diabetes and hypertension and trauma are often causes in adults. In the aetiology of sixth nerve palsies, it is important to consider this at a number of levels, namely nuclear (including a number of congenital disorders), fascicular (infarction, demyelination and tumour), subarachnoid (vascular, infective, tumours), petrous temporal (infection, sinus thrombosis and trauma), cavernous sinus and superior orbital fissure (vascular causes from internal carotid aneurysm, dissection,

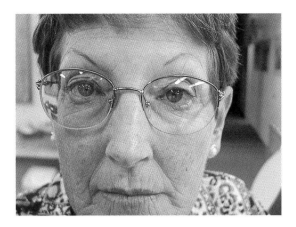

Figure 5.2   A long-standing left sixth nerve palsy associated with hypertension, development of cataract and reduced vision from 6/12 to 6/60

pituitary fossa tumour, Tolosa–Hunt syndrome) (Figure 5.2).

Other causes of adult strabismus

Convergence insufficiency

Diplopia at near due to convergence difficulty may be seen in patients following head trauma, Parkinson disease or Huntington disease.

Skew deviation

Differential diagnosis of inferior oblique overaction is a skew deviation. Skew deviation is a vertical deviation that cannot be isolated to a single extraocular muscle. It is almost always associated with other manifestations of the posterior fossa disease.

Acute diplopia in adults

Vertical diplopia of sudden onset in the adult includes the need to consider thyroid eye disease, myasthenia gravis, third and fourth nerve palsy and, rarely, myositis, on the background of microvascular disease such as diabetes or hypertension. In older patients, Steel-Richardson syndrome and giant cell arteritis may also be an important consideration.

Fourth nerve palsy is common and the majority of cases are congenital or traumatic. The patient may not be aware of compensatory head postures, but old photos will confirm. If the superior oblique palsy is not congenital or traumatic, a neurological consultation to exclude intracranial neoplasm is mandatory.

Horizontal diplopia is usually related to sixth nerve paresis and is obvious clinically. Trauma, vascular disease and raised intracranial pressure are the commonest causes. Diplopia in the older person is sometimes ascribed to divergence insufficiency. There may be associated symptoms of nystagmus, vertigo or dizziness on head turn, suggesting vertebrobasilar insufficiency. The diplopia is often readily corrected with prisms and may reflect underlying bilateral mild sixth nerve palsy. It is important to consider whether or not to investigate carotid and vertebral circulations and the associated circle of Willis depending on the patient's age and possibility of therapeutic intervention.

Horizontal diplopia may occur as a result of a lesion in the medial longitudinal fasciculus due to multiple sclerosis in a young adult or micro-vascular disease in the older patient. An important cause to consider is internuclear ophthalmoplegia. The leading eye will reveal abducting nystagmus, whilst the following eye will show inability to adduct in horizontal gaze in the presence of diplopia, and convergence is usually preserved. A diverse range of disease processes can damage the sixth nerve causing horizontal diplopia, reflecting its long course from the brainstem to the lateral rectus.

References

1. Calcutt C, Murray AD. Untreated essential infantile esotropia: factors affecting the development of amblyopia. *Eye* 1998;**12**:167–72.
2. Calcutt C. The natural history of infantile esotropia. A study of the untreated condition in the visual adult. *Advances in Amblyopia and Strabismus*. Transactions of the VIIth International Orthoptic Congress, Nurnberg, 1991.
3. Pratt-Johnson JA. 18th Annual Frank Costenbader Lecture. Fusion and suppression: development and loss. *J Pediatr Ophthalmol Strabismus* 1992;**29**:4–11.
4. Pratt-Johnson JA, Tillson G. Suppression in strabismus – an update. *Br J Ophthalmol* 1984;**68**:174–8.
5. Pratt-Johnson JA, Tillson G, Pop A. Suppression in strabismus and the hemiretinal trigger mechanism. *Arch Ophthalmol* 1983;**101**:218–24.
6. Parks MM. Isolated cyclovertical muscle palsy. *Arch Ophthalmol* 1958;**60**:1027–35.
7. Guyton DL. Exaggerated traction test for the oblique muscles. *Ophthalmology* 1981;**88**:1035–40.
8. Rootman J. *Diseases of the Orbit*. Philadelphia: J.B. Lippincott, 1988.

Section III
Management of strabismus

6 Assessment of strabismus

This chapter includes key points to consider in history taking and outlines a basic approach to assessing visual acuity and eye movements in preverbal children and adults. In preverbal children most reliance is placed on motor tests and observation. In the older child and adult sensory tests are complementary to motor tests.

The infant and preverbal child

Whilst a history is being taken, the child should be left undisturbed in a stroller, or the older child be allowed to play with toys. It is better if the doctor is not wearing a white coat or other trappings of the profession. An atmosphere of friendliness should be nurtured and the examination should be fun and, as far as possible, be an extension of a game. More can be gained from informality than from formality with children.

Vision in the newborn and developing infant excites the curiosity of a child to explore their environment, integrated with neck and general body movement. The visual interest that a child has in its environment will be strongly influenced by the child's intelligence and attentiveness.

The assessment and examination of the oculomotor system must be a reflection of both eye movements and visual function, both monocular and binocular. Strabismus that has its onset in childhood is particularly important because of the association between strabismus and amblyopia. Assessment and management of amblyopia is discussed in Chapter 7.

History

In addition to an account of the parent's perception of their child's strabismus, it is important to ask who first observed the strabismus and the observations they made. It is also important to take great care in determining the child's general health and development. Open-ended questions are important in focusing upon the problems of most concern to the parents. Where vision is at risk, careful questions about hearing should also be made. For example, what is the child's response to the sound of the telephone or a knock at the door? As vision strongly excites a child's interest, apparent delay in motor development may be a clue for visual impairment.

Other questions should include enquiry about the pregnancy, occurrence of rash, fevers, medications and drug abuse including alcohol, particularly in the early months of pregnancy. Family history should also be taken regarding eye movement disorders, but also hereditary visual defects, such as retinitis pigmentosa. Questions about the child's vision and how this compares to other children of similar age or siblings at the same age may also be helpful.

History and examination of a child with a squint should seek to establish that:

- the underlying cause of the strabismus is static; either monocular or binocular

- the vision in each eye is normal and equal

- the pattern of the abnormal eye movement is constant at a particular test distance.

The underlying cause may be progressive, for example chiasmal glioma[1] (see Figure 4.12), or non-progressive, for example some forms of rod monochromatism. It is important to detect the defect in vision, to recognise that the strabismus is secondary to pathology and to determine that the child's vision is abnormal. It is not uncommon for the visual deterioration in preverbal children with craniopharyngioma or optic nerve glioma to go undetected until later. In these cases, often more attention is given to the eye movement disorder than the defect in vision and occasionally eyes are operated on without recognising the underlying visual defect until later. It is equally important to distinguish the presence of a pseudosquint, most commonly due to the configuration of the eyelids, particularly epicanthal folds, creating an optical illusion (Figure 6.1). It is important to bear in mind that a true deviation of one eye may be apparent at the same time as visual axis alignment. In such cases normal binocular vision is present. This may be due to heterotopia of the macula, occasionally seen in children who have had retinopathy of prematurity, to exclude retinal pathology. Epicanthal folds have different significance with relation to race and presence of developmental disorders. A diagnosis of pseudosquint can be made only after the exclusion of true strabismus, which may coexist with epicanthal folds. Other clinical features should be looked for which may give clues to an underlying cause of epicanthal folds and strabismus, for example Down syndrome (Figure 6.2).

It is important to determine whether the parents have noticed inattention to the visual field of either side, rubbing of the eyes (oculodigital reflex), or whether the child makes eye contact or is fascinated by mobiles over the cot. A child's disinterest in a visual object can reflect intellectual delay.

In the older child, it must be determined whether the child prefers to be in dull or bright

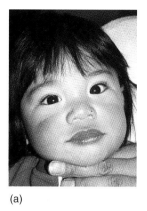 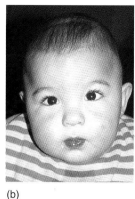

(a) (b)

Figure 6.1 Epicanthial folds in children (a, b) giving rise to the appearance of pseudostrabismus

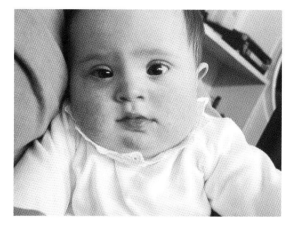

Figure 6.2 In a younger baby, milder forms of syndromes, e.g. Down syndrome, may be missed. In this case there was an associated central cataract typical of Down syndrome in addition to epicanthal folds. Cataracts were removed in the first week of life and contact lenses fitted. Children such as these and premature infants need to be assessed carefully and monitored for development of subsequent strabismus

light, and whether the child becomes frightened in the dark and seeks to hold onto parents. Marked intolerance of bright light may indicate rod monochromatism, in which case the child may behave as if totally blind in bright light. Such a case may also present with esotropia and nystagmus and needs consideration as a case of congenital esotropia. It is important to ask how close the child holds toys to examine them, and what is the child's behaviour with the television.

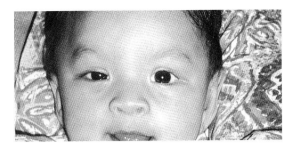

Figure 6.3 The eyelid configuration and position may present as pseudosquint particularly in respect to epicanthal folds. The presence of ptosis should lead to a careful appraisal of the superior rectus muscle which may also be underdeveloped. Note the mild dextroversion of the eyes giving an impression of small left convergent squint

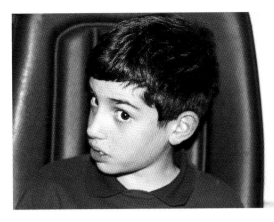

Figure 6.4 Abnormal head posture (AHP) in a child with congenital nystagmus. The abnormal head posture may not be obvious initially in examination as visual acuity is tested. With smaller targets presented, the AHP may increase in order to reach the null point of fixation and increase the foveation time

For example, does he or she prefer to be almost touching the screen?

Clinical examination

The cooperation and trust of children are essential in any clinical examination. The success of the examination is said to commence from the moment the child enters the ophthalmologist's consulting rooms. It helps if the child is seen amongst other children, that the clinic staff are friendly and get on well with children, and that within the rooms there are areas set aside for play.

If the child is distressed it is important to make certain that the parents are at ease. Giving the child toys to play with and concentrating on the parents and gaining their confidence quickly translates into an examination with a cooperative child. Much can be learned by watching the children play and how they move their eyes from the moment they enter the consulting room.

In infancy and the preverbal child, the qualities of vision are often inferred from motor responses. When assessing movement and the eye's ability to see and follow the object, it is important not to give auditory clues.

It is important to observe the presence of strabismus, nystagmus or abnormal head posture. Abnormal head posture (AHP) (Figure 6.4) may

be maintained to avoid double vision or to improve visual acuity (for example, in Ciancia syndrome) or to centre the visual field. Manifest deviation should be tested quickly so as not to disrupt binocular vision. Where there is no obvious squint it is wise to assess binocular vision, fusion and stereopsis before assessment. In the absence of binocular vision it is essential to determine the dominant eye; this is not always easy in an uncooperative child. AHP in strabismus can result from preferred fixation with the eye with restricted movement since infancy. The child may prefer to fix with the eye with restricted movement and adopt an abnormal head posture to best exploit his or her visual field in that eye. Such cases are also seen in Moebius syndrome or where torsion has been a complication of surgery to the fixing eye in strabismus.

Among children referred with AHP and strabismus fixus affecting one eye there has been a failure to appreciate that the eye with abnormal movement was the fixing eye, leading to advice to patch the eye, with full movement making the vision worse in that eye where vision was already compromised.

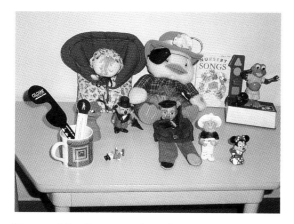

Figure 6.5 An example of toys useful in the examination of young children

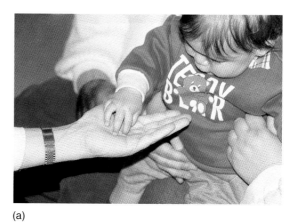

(a)

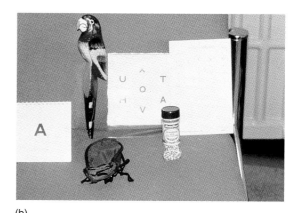

(b)

Figure 6.6 Testing of fixation of small targets. (a) Note child adopting pincer movement to pick up cake decoration from examiner's hand. (b) Note fixation and target matching and bottle of cake decorations

Tests of visual acuity

These should be performed preferably at distance and near, both monocularly and binocularly with appropriate refractive correction.

Fixation

It is important to observe whether fixation is central, steady and maintained, both monocularly and binocularly. If fixation is not monocular, it is suggestive of a visual defect and a risk factor for strabismus. This may be further confirmed if the child is happy with one eye occluded and not the other. Children need small detailed toys for near and larger animated toys or pictures at distance. It is useful to provide a range of toys for such examination (Figure 6.5). The ability of each eye to maintain fixation in a freely alternating fashion suggests equal vision. Although the eyes may not alternate fixation freely, sustaining fixation may be observed to vary from complete inability to longer periods before reverting back to fixation with the dominant eye, indicating useful vision.

Fixation and following

The ability of an infant to fix and follow can be simply tested. Fixation should be steady and should be accompanied by smooth pursuit movements. No auditory signal should be given at

the time of the test. Occlusion of one eye may be distressing if vision is poor in the unoccluded eye.

Fixation of small targets

Having been given a taste for cake decorations ("hundreds and thousands"), the infant is presented with one cake decoration in the palm of the examiner's hand (Figure 6.6). The examiner observes the child to see whether the child picks up the object with a pincer grip with the finger and thumb, which indicates good vision, or a raking movement, for example in a 1-year old child. Raking movements indicate poor vision. Using the pincer movement to pick up single hundreds and thousands indicates not only good vision but good hand–eye coordination.

Teller acuity cards and forced preferential looking

In the preverbal child, the forced preferential looking depends on the child's inherent interest in patterns as opposed to other targets. Here the child is observed through a small hole and various grating sizes are presented and the child's response noted.[2,3,4] Teller acuity cards consist of cards with varying sizes of vertical gratings (see Figure 2.3). They are useful for assessing the vision of the preverbal child as well as the ability to maintain and hold fixation.[5,6] They may also be particularly helpful in comparing the vision between the two eyes although they overestimate visual acuity in amblyopia.

Matching tests

Matching tests such as the E test, Sheridan–Gardiner and Mackay tests may be used in children as young as 2–3 years. Other picture matching card tests may also be useful. In the very small child cooperation is better if the test is performed at a distance of one third of a metre.

Poor vision testing

Useful tests particularly in preverbal children suspected of poor vision include:

- *Optokinetic nystagmus induced with optokinetic tape.* The tape is passed in front of the child's eyes and the nystagmus made up of refixation pursuit episodes is observed.

- *Vestibulo-ocular reflex test.* The examiner rotates with the child held at arms length and facing the examiner which induces horizontal nystagmus. After cessation of rotation it is noted how quickly the vestibulo-ocular reflex is overridden by the visual fixation reflex as the child takes up visual fixation on the examiner's face. If nystagmus is prolonged, it suggests that the baby is blind or has severe cerebellar disease.

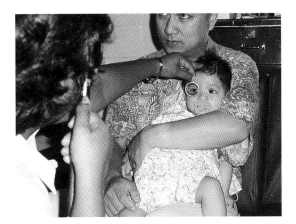

Figure 6.7   Cycloplegic refraction of a young child

Occlusion

The use of an occluder card or paddle is often preferable to ensure that an eye is properly occluded, although using a thumb may often be as efficient.

Refractive error

It is important to perform full cycloplegic retinoscopy on the child in order to determine the degree of refractive error present in each eye, which may contribute to strabismus and subsequent amblyopia. Instillation of cycloplegic drops 2 days prior to examination ensures adequate effect; however, it is important to warn parents of possible systemic side effects (Figure 6.7).

Colour vision

Ishihara plates are useful, although they only test red–green deficiency. The test may be simplified by asking the child to trace the coloured path with a finger. Errors that do not conform to red–green deficiency may indicate optic nerve disease.

Pupil

Examination of the pupil may give information about the optic nerve and the third cranial nerve.

Sensory evaluation – binocular vision, fusion, and stereopsis

Tests of binocular vision are important not only to exclude strabismus, but also to assess the extent of visual impairment.

Stereopsis

In children, the Titmus Fly and the Lang tests are useful determinants of stereopsis. High grade stereopsis implies good visual acuity in both eyes and some degree of fusion. Poor stereopsis may occur with poor monocular vision in each eye or diminished acuity in either or both eyes.[7] The Titmus Fly test is widely used and uses dissociation polaroid glasses. There is a larger representation of a house fly and smaller representations of animals and circles. The Lang test involves a random dot stereogram incorporated into a card and has the advantage that glasses need not be used. Other stereopsis tests include the TNO random dot stereopsis test.

Testing of monofixation syndromes

The testing of a stable strabismus angle with peripheral fusion and a monofixation syndrome (MFS) is important and is the result obtained in optimally treated congenital esotropia. The diagnosis of MFS requires evidence of absence of central binocular vision or bifoveal fixation and the presence of peripheral binocular vision and fusion.

The diagnosis of absence of bifoveal fixation requires the documentation of a macular scotoma.

- Firstly, useful and more commonly used tests include Bagolini striate glasses (see following section). In the presence of a microsquint, if there is peripheral fusion the patient will see a cross. If the patient has sufficient cognitive maturity, they may be able to describe the scotoma.

- Secondly, the AO vectograph project-O chart slide has value in documenting the facultative scotoma of MFS. Patients with MFS delete letters that image in the eye with the fixation scotoma.

- Thirdly the testing of stereoacuity provides useful evidence of gross stereopsis indicating peripheral fusion and about 200–300 seconds of arc of stereopsis. Fine stereopsis of more than 40 seconds of arc implies the patient has bifoveal fixation. Another useful motor test for monofixation is the 4 D base out prism test (Figure 6.8). During binocular viewing, quickly introduce a 4 D base out prism. Both eyes will move away from the base of the prism – if binocular vision is normal, the eye not covered by the prism will make a corrective convergent movement. This response occurs no matter which eye the prism is placed over. By contrast in MFS, when the base out prism is introduced in front of the fixing eye, there is the movement of both eyes away from the base of the prism, but the eye with MFS does not take up free fixation. If the prism is placed in front of the non-fixing eye, there may be no movement. Occasionally MFS causes a switch fixation each time the prism is moved. This test is probably the least reliable to diagnose the presence of macular scotoma.[8]

Fusion

Worth 4-dot test Fusion tests include the Worth 4-dot test involving four illuminated dots arranged in a diamond with the red above and the white below and two horizontal green dots between and lateral to these (Figure 6.9). The four dots are viewed through red and green glasses that are complementary to the illuminated colours. When fusion is present, four dots are seen, with the white dot changing colour due to retinal rivalry. If diplopia is present, five dots will be seen. If suppression is present, the child will see two or three. The test has been criticised because the artificial need to wear green and red filters breaks down phorias and because the test underestimates in some people.

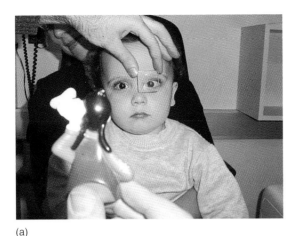

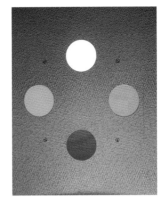

Figure 6.9   The Worth 4-dot test for fusion

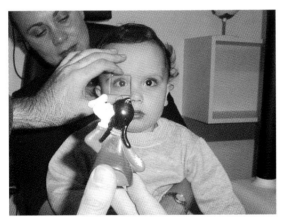

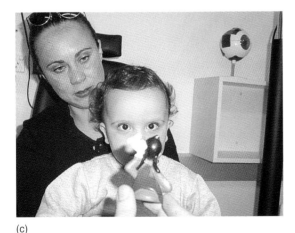

Figure 6.8   The 4 D base out prism test providing supporting evidence of normal binocular vision. When the prism is interposed to maintain binocular vision, the eye subjected to the prism makes a convergent movement while the other eye maintains fixation

Bagolini striate glasses   A test that comes closest to the natural environment and testing in free space is that using Bagolini lenses. The lenses are striated with each eye at right angles to the other, so a pinpoint of light will be seen as a cross (Figure 6.10). As the test is done in free space, the patient is aware of peripheral objects surrounding the light which optimise the association between the two eyes, allowing the most natural environment for testing. In MFS, the fovea of the non-dominant eye is suppressed under non-binocular conditions. The cross is seen because of peripheral fusion. The patient's interpretation of what is seen gives an indication of the state of fusion. If the patients are mature enough, they may be asked to draw what they see and Figure 6.10 shows some of the more common representations that the patient will draw. In normal retinal correspondence, MFS is a condition where there is suppression of one fovea under binocular viewing. The condition may be primary and without strabismus, although it is more commonly associated with a small angle strabismus which is usually convergent but may be divergent.

Amblyoscope or synoptophore   The use of this instrument now figures less in orthoptic practice than previously. It has value particularly in large angle squint, giving some indication of fusion and the capacity to build upon this.

63

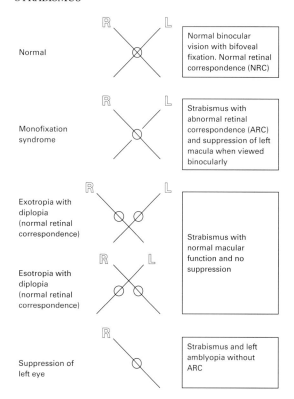

Figure 6.10 Bagolini striated glasses consist of two plano lenses (one for each eye) with parallel striations for one eye set at right angles to the striations for the other. The patient views a light at 6 m through the glasses. If there is normal binocular vision the light is perceived as two lines at right angles to each other passing through the centre of each other. As the test is done in free space, the patient is aware of peripheral objects surrounding the light which optimise the association between the two eyes, allowing the most natural environment for testing. In MFS, the fovea of the non-dominant eye is suppressed under binocular conditions. The cross is seen because of peripheral fusion

Motor evaluation – eye movements and alignment

Hirschberg corneal light reflex test

Estimation of the corneal light reflex is one of the simplest tests of ocular alignment. When testing the corneal light reflex both the source of light and the target should be held together. A small nasal displacement of the corneal light reflex is not uncommon in young children (Figure 6.11).

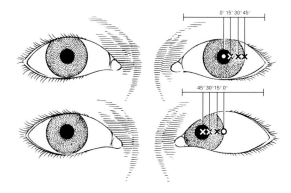

Figure 6.11 The Hirschberg corneal light reflex test

Krimsky test

The Krimsky test uses a prism bar to equalise the position of the light reflex from each eye; half the number of prism dioptres of the deviation equals magnitude of the deviation in degrees (Figure 6.12).

Bruckner test

This test determines the presence of a strabismus in the uncooperative child who may not tolerate cover tests. A test light beam is held at 1 m and the brightness of the red reflex in each eye is compared. If the red reflex is brighter in one eye than the other, then it is likely that strabismus is present in the eye with the brighter reflex. The disturbance of the accommodation component of the near reflex raises a doubt that the Bruckner test can be relied upon under 2 months of age. The reason lies in the smaller pupil and poorer central vision in newborns who have a greater depth of focus than adults, and as accommodation does not need to be as exact, this in turn affects the accuracy of the test. We have found that it is useful after the age of 4 months but it has been argued that it is not completely reliable until after 8 months.[9]

15 D base out prism test

The 15 D base out prism test is a useful test in infants. It stresses the binocular fusion by

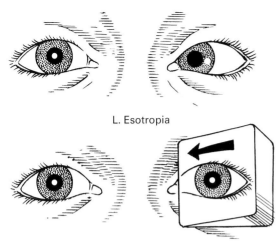

L. Esotropia

Measured with prism & light reflex

Note: If left eye is blind place prism in front of the
sighted right eye.
Power of prism to align is measurement in
prism dioptres.
Can measure in 9 cardinal positions.

Figure 6.12   The Krimsky light reflex test

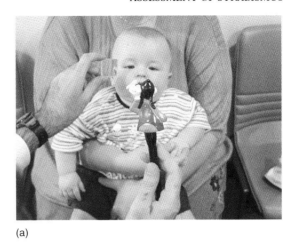

(a)

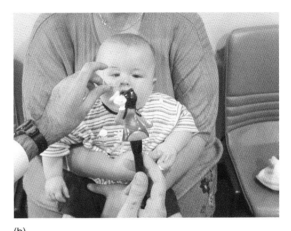

(b)

Figure 6.13   The 15 D base out prism test. A
fixation toy is used as a target and corrective eye
movements are observed in response to a 15 dioptre
base out prism challenge

shifting the retinal image and observing the
motor response convergence in the eye with the
base out prism and recovery of alignment on
removal of the prism. Overcoming a 15 D base
out prism is an indicator of fusion ability and
may be a helpful quick screening test in infants
and young children (Figure 6.13).

Cover tests

Cover tests demand control of fixation and
cooperation of the child. They should be
performed for near and distance fixation and
provide both sensory and motor information.
They should be performed with the patient
wearing optical correction.

The monocular cover–uncover test differen-
tiates a phoria (latent squint) from a tropia
(manifest squint). The alternate cover test
measures the total deviation, both latent (phoria)
and manifest (tropia). Following dissociation, the
deviation can be measured using a simultaneous
prism–cover test to determine the actual deviation
when both eyes are uncovered.

4 D base out prism test

Microsquints difficult to detect with traditional cover tests may be diagnosed with the 4 D
base out prism test (see above).[10]

Maddox rod

The Maddox rod test dissociates the two
eyes. The device creates a vertical line from a
point light source; one eye will view the point
light source, the other a vertical line. Since
fusion is produced, the test can be used for
horizontal and vertical deviations. In addition,

torsional deviations can be measured using another Maddox rod.

Saccade velocity and pursuit

The examination is not complete without examining for saccades and pursuit, and being alert to the possibility of internuclear ophthalmoplegia, oculomotor apraxia or progressive external ophthalmoplegia. The examiner with experience rapidly learns to recognise normal and abnormal pursuit.

Assessment of abnormal head posture

Measurements of deviation are made in the primary position and in all positions of gaze. This is important for two main reasons:

- determining the basis of abnormal head positions, and
- detection of incomitant squints associated with cranial nerve palsies as well as A and V patterns.

The examination provides information about third, fourth, and sixth cranial nerves together with supranuclear control of eye movement.

The differential diagnosis of abnormal head posture includes:

- causes of torticollis, including hemivertebra, sternomastoid tumour or monoaural deafness
- ocular causes, including nystagmus, fourth nerve palsy, and homonymous hemianopia.

Assessment of paretic strabismus

Useful information can be obtained by the clinician via a number of simple tests.

Head tilt

If head tilt has been assumed to maintain binocular vision and avoid diplopia, a cover test with the head in the tilted position will demonstrate that the eyes are straight and that fusion is probably present. It can be tested also by simple tests of fusion, including the Lang test. Having taken visual acuity, the head can be tilted to the opposite side to see if this disrupts fusion.

Diplopia test

If it is on the basis of binocular imbalance, one image will disappear on occlusion of either eye. The angle of deviation will be greatest in the deviation of the paretic muscle when the eye is fixing with the paretic muscle (Hering's Law). This test is of more use in the older child or adult. Dissociating the eyes with red and green glasses may assist evaluation.

Diplopia tests may be helpful in several scenarios, including facilitating the diagnosis of a horizontal muscle palsy; for example, in a left sixth nerve paresis, the diplopia and deviation will be greatest in the direction of the left lateral rectus. Cyclovertical muscle imbalance may be determined by direct observation of the patient or by questioning. The Parks 3-step test may be used both subjectively as well as objectively (see Chapter 5). The patient may be asked the following questions.

- In which eye is the image higher?
- Whether vertical separation is wider on head tilt to the left or right.
- Whether vertical separation is greater on right or left gaze.

This information is sufficient to make the presumptive diagnosis as to which cyclovertical muscle is involved.

The pointer test

A useful diagnostic test to confirm diagnosis of a fourth nerve palsy is the pointer test (Figure 6.14).

Plotting ocular posture

The Hess chart, Lees screen or Foster screen tests can be initiated by suppression or

PATIENT VIEWS POINTER HELD IN LOWER FIELD
BY EXAMINER.

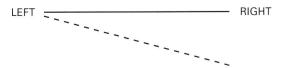

ANGLE FORMED BY FALSE IMAGE AND TRUE
IMAGE POINTS TO SIDE OF PARESIS.

Figure 6.14   The pointer test

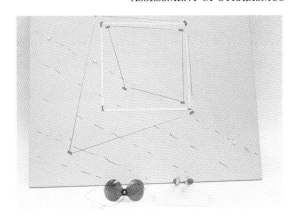

Figure 6.15   The Foster test. Note the underaction of the right superior oblique muscle and the overaction of the synergistic left inferior rectus

alternation. These tests are useful to establish a baseline and compare progress. The Hess tangent screen plots the relative position of each eye (posture) in nine positions of gaze. The patient wears complementary red and green goggles to disassociate the eyes and the test is done at 50 cm. The screen has small red lights that can be illuminated. The patient holds a green light and attempts to place it on the illuminated red light. The eye with the red goggle views the red light and is the fixing eye. The eye with the green goggle is the eye in which the posture is being studied. The Lees screen and Foster screen are variants of this test. The Foster screen is a simple inexpensive test that can be easily made (Figure 6.15). Note that further objective information about the paretic muscle can be obtained by measuring the deviation in prisms in the direction of action of the affected muscle.

Determining muscle restriction or paresis

Determining whether a muscle is restricted or paretic may be based on observation of eye movements. In the paretic eye, there will be slowing of saccades. In the eye with mechanical restriction (for example, muscle entrapment) the velocity of saccade is normal until movement ceases with the restriction.

Restriction – forced duction test   The eye is anaesthetised with a cotton bud soaked with 4% lignocaine (or cocaine). Fine toothed forceps

hold the globe. The patient is asked to look in the direction of the muscle under investigation. The eye is then moved in that direction. In the eye with the paretic muscle it will be possible to extend the movement, whereas restriction will be experienced as resistance to movement. In children under 12 years, the case should be done in theatre under anaesthetic prior to the commencement of strabismus surgery. In our experience, the eye should be kept in the position of primary action although others believe the muscles should be pushed or lifted up.[11] The test is only useful if obviously positive.

Paresis – active force generation test
The eye is grasped with forceps after instilling the area with anaesthetic on a cotton bud tip and the patient is asked to move the eye in the primary direction of action. For example, in a lateral rectus palsy the globe is grasped medially whilst the patient attempts to adduct the eye and the amount of force generated is noted.

Assessment in the older child and the adult

The techniques of assessment in preverbal children are applicable to the older child and

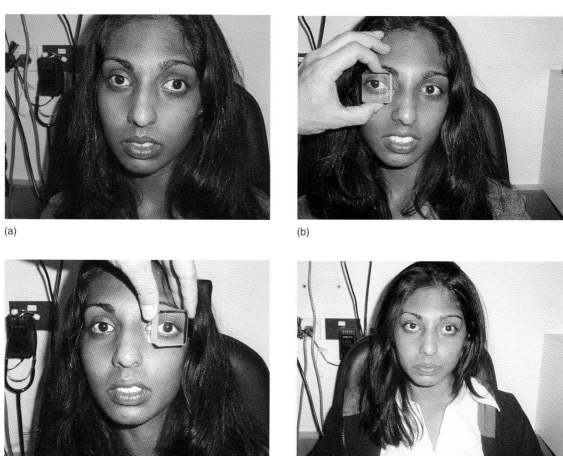

(a)

(b)

(c)

(d)

Figure 6.16   Prism estimation of strabismus deviation. The divergent left eye was amblyopic from an injury in childhood which damaged the macula. An appropriate prism in front of the fixing eye allows an assessment of the amount of deviation consistent with Hering's Law in contrast to the prism in front of the amblyopic eye (a-c). (d) shows good cosmetic result following surgical correction

adults. Additional information may be obtained in the adult because of greater cooperation, particularly with diplopia tests, and forced duction and force generation tests can be carried out in the clinic without resorting to the need for general anaesthesia.

In a comprehensive approach to the adult patient suggestive of oculomotor dysfunction, it is important that the examination take account of a number of features, particularly about the head and neck, that give clues to the oculomotor system in strabismus in particular.

Head and neck features

- *Postures*: abnormal head posture (AHP) (see Figure 4.18), tilts, turns, chin up or down, head tremors and head thrusting on refixation, features of naevus flammeus.

- *Lid position with eye movements*: palpebral aperture changes with eye movements.

Detailed visual examination

Visual acuity, visual field and pupillary responses.

Saccades

Note saccades in response to auditory or visual targets, for example clicking fingers in different areas of field, noting velocity, accuracy, latency and the working together of the eyes. Assessment of the quick phase by using an optokinetic tape. This also gives information about pursuit and refixation.

Smooth pursuit and range of eye movements

Test the patient's ability to smoothly track a moving object, carrying out versions with both eyes open and ductions with one eye open. The range of eye movements is usually tested by asking the patient to follow the target into the nine positions of gaze.

Vergence

Testing vergence binocularity with 15 D base out prism, vergence with accommodation, convergence recovery, noting papillary response along the mid-sagittal plane in the primary position (bearing in mind light–near dissociation of pupil responses).

Cover tests for ocular alignment

- Cover tests measuring deviation, with accommodation controlled with the patient wearing the correct glasses (an accurate and thorough assessment of ocular alignment is more meaningful when the full optical correction is worn).
- Measurement of the strabismic angle using the prism cover test (Figure 6.16).

Vestibular function

Measure acuity when shaking the patient's head to see if this degrades the visual acuity.

References

1. Billson F. Tumours of the eye and orbit. In: Jones PC, Campbell PE, eds. *Tumours of Infancy and Childhood*. Oxford: Blackwell Scientific Publications, 1976: 397–440.
2. Fulton AB, Hanson RM, Manning KA. Measuring visual acuity in infants. *Surv Ophthalmol* 1981;**25**: 325–32.
3. Jacobson SG, Mohindra I, Held R. Visual acuity of infants with ocular disease. *Am J Ophthalmol* 1982; **93**:198–209.
4. Catalano R, Simon J, Jenkins P, Kandel G. Preferential looking as a guide for amblyopia therapy in infantile cataracts. *J Paediatr Ophthalmol Strabismus* 1987;**24**: 56–63.
5. Dobson V, Teller DY. Visual acuity in human infants: a review and comparison of behavioral and electrophysiological studies. *Vision Res* 1978;**18**: 1469–83.
6. Teller D. Visual acuity for vertical and diagonal gratings in human infants. *Vision Res* 1974;**14**:1433–9.
7. Donzis P, Rapazzo J, Burde R, Gordon M. Effect of binocular variations of Snellen's visual acuity on Titmus stereoacuity. *Arch Ophthalmol* 1983;**101**:930–2.
8. Lang J. Evaluation of small angle strabismus or microtropia. In: Aruga A, ed. *Strabismus Symposium*. Basel: Karger, 1968.
9. Archer SM. Developmental aspect of the Bruckner Test. *Ophthalmology* 1988;**95**:1098.
10. Jampolsky A. The prism test for strabismus screening. *J Paediatr Ophthalmol Strabismus* 1964;**1**:30–3.
11. Guyton DL. Exaggerated traction test for the oblique muscles. *Ophthalmology* 1981;**88**:1035–40.

7 Therapy of strabismus

Non-surgical therapy

The team approach to strabismus

In the unravelling of strabismus and eye movement disorders, the ophthalmologist and the eye health professional team form the nucleus for the investigation of the ocular motor system. However, it is essential that they see themselves also as a part of a larger team where the child is the centre of focus. In children, eye movement disorders may rarely be part of systemic or neurologic system disorders and at times they may require the expert advice of geneticists, radiologists, neurologists, dysmorphologists and good paediatricians both specialist and general, with team members all working closely with the family and the family doctor. This is particularly important in a children's hospital where so often the consultation is about a child or infant in the care of another colleague. By contrast, outside of the hospital setting, ophthalmologists, family doctors, and community eye care workers may be the first point of contact and it is important that they understand child and visual development and recognise what may appear to be "a simple squint" but is in fact a clinical sign of underlying disease requiring further investigation.

Eye health professionals can and do play a valuable role in the recognition and care of the strabismic child and in working closely with the ophthalmologist. However, potentially the most valuable members of this team are the parents. Other trusted adults in the child's life including teachers can also play an important role.

The parents as part of the team

Time should be spent with the parents to explain in simple terms the natural history of the particular form of strabismus the child has. Time should be spent explaining the concept of amblyopia and how each eye "competes for visual space in the brain" and how the constantly squinting eye may not gain equal visual space and as a result lose sight and become amblyopic. It must be made clear that surgical alignment does not improve vision; indeed it increases the need for vigilance and continued intermittent occlusion. Occlusion treatment should be explained and the risk of occlusion amblyopia.

Time should be spent explaining the importance of visual tasks during occlusion; for example in a young uncooperative child the mother can be advised to supervise occlusion while the meal is prepared. The other children are excluded from the room and the child is given the opportunity to colour in pictures or do simple tasks with toy blocks, puzzles or hand held electronic games. It should be explained that the younger the infant, the more rapidly vision is lost from amblyopia, the more rapidly it can be recovered and that occlusion amblyopia can occur more quickly in the infant and young child than in the older child.

Total occlusion is easier to control in younger children. Arm splints prevent the child from removing the occlusion but leave the hands free for the child to play (Figure 7.1). If the child is

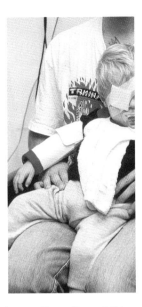

Figure 7.1 Arm splints allow child to play but not remove patch

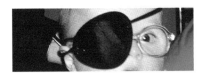

Figure 7.2 Black pirate patch. Can alternatively be attached to glasses

long sighted and requires glasses to control the squint but refuses to wear glasses, initial use of mydriatic drops daily will make the vision blurred without glasses. In this circumstance acceptance of glasses is made easier.

Some young children enjoy wearing an eye patch if they feel they're playing a character like a pirate (Figure 7.2). School-age children can be unkind about difference, calling children with glasses "four-eyes", calling children with squint "dumb". We've even known children to refuse to sit with children with visual problems. In kindergarten children are more accepting, and kindergarten teachers can do much to explain and assist the child receiving treatment. From age 6 onwards it becomes more difficult with larger classes and students are more difficult to control. In some cases children won't wear glasses, but more frequently they flatly refuse to wear occlusion. In such cases it is our strongly held belief that occlusion should be part time and carried on out of school hours.

With this regime we have plenty of experience of recovery of vision, including amongst children brought for second opinion because of refusal to accept occlusion during school hours. In young and also older children, the near vision test charts matching tests can be photocopied and parents encouraged to check progress of the occlusion tests at home. Even the letters in the phone book can be used. Children wearing glasses often object to occlusion if the occluder is stuck to the face. This can be avoided by the use of paper occluders attached to the glasses.

With adults, the eye health professional team is smaller. The strabismus specialist treating the adult may not need an assistant because the adult should be more in control of their anxieties and should be more cooperative. However, unlike children, they may be demanding in a different way, depending on their expectations. They may seek cosmetic improvement, relief of double vision or seek restoration of binocular vision when this has been absent since childhood. Recent onset of symptoms in strabismus present since childhood are unlikely to be related unless there is decompensation, for example in a case of superior oblique paresis that has previously been fusing.

Management of amblyopia in strabismus

Management of strabismic amblyopia is a critical part of care of the strabismic infant or child. Strabismic amblyopia has a critical period more extended than in pattern deprivation amblyopia, though less than that in refractive amblyopia. It occurs during development when there is plasticity of the brain. Simple occlusion of the eye with good vision will allow the amblyopic eye to recover vision. Indeed, if occlusion is prolonged the occluded eye becomes amblyopic. This reversal of amblyopia is referred to as occlusion amblyopia. It is important also to recognise and treat the other forms of amblyopia, namely pattern and anisometropic, which may also contribute to the poor vision.

Arising from the above are the three principles of management that should be followed before surgery is considered:

- confirming that the amblyopia is strabismic in type

- ensuring an accurate refraction for each eye, and

- ensuring occlusion therapy with a regime appropriate to each individual case.

These three principles and the exclusion of central nervous system or ocular pathology are essential to observe before any consideration is given to strabismus surgery.

Principles and strategies for non-surgical therapy of strabismus and amblyopia

Confirming strabismic amblyopia

Careful examination and refraction will usually allow confirmation of the nature of the amblyopia. However, unilateral optic nerve hypoplasia is a pathological lesion sometimes missed, the halo around the small disc being mistaken for the neural rim. Posterior lenticonus may be missed early and as it is frequently followed by the development of progressive cataract in infancy, it may contribute to a pattern deprivation amblyopia. If there is doubt the matter is usually readily resolved with the additional information from examination under anaesthetic, including biomicroscopy and confirming refraction.

Confirming refraction

As pointed out in the text referring to assessment (see Chapter 6), it is essential to gain the trust of the child and the parent. Staff should not be in white coats. Eye drops may be a frightening experience for the child. With a particularly anxious and frightened child, there may be wisdom in writing a prescription for atropine 0·5% or 1% eye drops depending on the age of the child and instructing the parents how to instil the drops morning and night two days before the visit and on the morning of the visit. However, parents should be warned that reactions may occur in the form of irritability, flushing and raised temperature, particularly in the very young and more often in children with cerebral palsy or impaired temperature control.

Prescription of glasses

No child or infant is too young to wear glasses. The decision to order glasses is frequently sufficient for some parents to seek a second opinion, so it is important to spend time speaking to the parents so that they understand the underlying reasons. In the premature infant glasses are usually deferred at least until corrected age is about term. Our experience is that in the early period of life, particularly in infants born prematurely, there are changes toward emmetropisation that justify watching carefully to see if refraction is stabilising before ordering glasses. Prescription of glasses to correct hypermetropia in an accommodative strabismus is usually in the second or third year of life. Less commonly, hypermetropia may be among the spectrum of presentations of congenital esotropia.

Clinical tips

It is important to remember that smaller degrees of hypermetropia prescribed after surgery for congenital esotropia may be effective in correction of residual deviations.

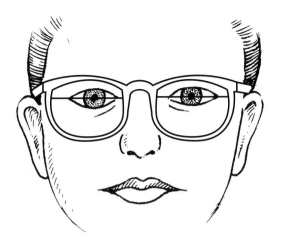

Figure 7.3 Accommodative strabismus with convergence excess. Executive bifocal glasses may assist control. Note the junction of the bifocals horizontally "splits" the pupil

- As a "rule of thumb", astigmatism, particularly if more than 2 D, is significant enough to be amblyogenic and, if unilateral, could be an asymmetrising factor in the development of strabismus.

- Children who are sufficiently myopic to justify ordering glasses may reveal accommodative strabismus with convergence excess when wearing glasses, and may require surgery to control the deviation.

- Children with accommodative strabismus with convergence excess may be helped to control the strabismus by wearing executive bifocals. It is important that the ophthalmologist checks the glasses and ensures that the horizontal junction between reading segment and the distance lenses splits the pupil (Figure 7.3). The reason for this is that as soon as the child lowers the eyes to view a near object, the need to accommodate is obviated.

- Anisometropic amblyopia has a more prolonged critical period than pattern deprivation and strabismic amblyopia, and prognosis for improvement of vision can be good even if treatment started after the age of 7 years.

Occlusion

Constant occlusion of the dominant eye is still the most effective method of treating an amblyopic eye. With a history that dates back to the 18th century, it continues to be the preferred method. Recent results of penalisation confirm this. Understanding the sensitivity of the developing infant's visual system (see Chapter 2) demands that occlusion in infancy be closely monitored. Monitoring of eyes that have been amblyopic or are at risk of amblyopia should continue at least until the child's visual system has matured (usually at age 9–10 years). The earlier the amblyopia is detected and the younger the child or infant, the shorter must be the occlusion.

Types of occlusion Full-time occlusion is most easily implemented in the preverbal and preschool child. However, after the age of 4–5 years and particularly at school, children's peer groups tease and indeed the poorer vision in the amblyopic eye may make for learning problems. Although not as effective, part-time occlusion is well worth implementing in cases where constant occlusion is not tolerated or maintenance occlusion is required. As previously mentioned, in our experience in university clinics, children of school age are most often only submitted to occlusion out of school hours doing homework, or in the younger child given play tasks demanding attention to near detail. We have found even a half to one hour effective in maintaining vision and even improving vision that had been poor because of refusal to cooperate in full-time occlusion.

Sometimes, with treatment of amblyopia, the patient has refused to wear glasses. In those cases with high refractive error or astigmatism, the use of atropine in each eye once or twice a week has been useful in the encouragement of wearing glasses. Traditional occlusion and partial occlusion of a lens to obstruct vision in a particular direction of gaze, for example by translucent paper, may have advantages over other forms of non-surgical management such as optical penalisation or prisms. The viewed object is not altered in shape, size or localisation and the amblyopic eye, having a clearer image with acuity now exceeding the non-amblyopic eye, may continue to become less amblyopic.

Prisms and filters

Prisms may be helpful in treating patients with small amounts of deviation in the vertical or horizontal directions.[1,2] This intervention is more often helpful in adult strabismus, for example vertical diplopia in thyroid eye disease or a previously controlled decompensating superior oblique weakness.

Prisms can have a place in management of a partially recovered sixth nerve palsy. Plastic prisms incorporated into spectacles have limited value because of bulk beyond 5–6 prism dioptres. However, Fresnel prisms are an alternative as they are lightweight, can be high powered and stuck temporarily on a patient's spectacles. The bulk and weight of the prism is reduced by the Fresnel principle that combines multiple small prisms of identical refractive angle in place of a larger prism, oriented to correct deviation. A typical case is that of a 77-year-old lady with incomplete recovery of a traumatic sixth nerve palsy after 12 months. Although high powered prisms blur the image to some extent, in this case we incorporated a 30 D base out Fresnel prism, restoring comfortable binocular vision and enabling improved patient mobility and reading comfort (Figure 7.4).

Exercises

Orthoptic exercises are based on the principle of expansion of fusional vergences. Common indications for exercises include convergence insufficiency, intermittent exotropia of small amplitude and decompensating accommodative esotropia. Children under 3 years and with less than 3 dioptres of hypermetropia often have a

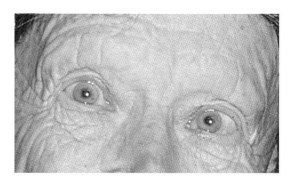

(a)

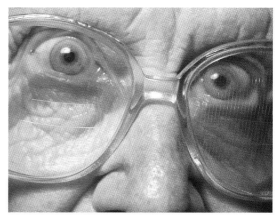

(b)

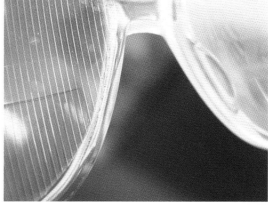

(c)

Figure 7.4   Older lady with post-traumatic residual left sixth nerve palsy (a) without glasses (b) after glasses with a Fresnel 20 dioptre prism pressed to the back of the left lens. (c) Detail of glasses (as viewed from the back), restoring binocular singular vision with adhesive Fresnel prisms base out

good chance of not wearing spectacles as adults. Older children with a low refractive error may also benefit from orthoptic exercises if the strabismus is fully controlled by optical correction.

Surgical therapy

Guidelines for surgical treatment of strabismus

It is important to take a careful history, to estimate visual acuity and to make measurements of the strabismus and determine what needs to be done. The decision must be shared with the parents. Time needs to be spent until the parents' expectations match the surgeon's. Equally important is the need to discuss with the parents the possibility of later development of other muscle imbalance including inferior oblique overaction and dissociated vertical deviation. The emergence of these after surgery may be seen by the parents as complications, if not explained to them beforehand. The principles of surgery must also consider both the horizontal and the vertical elements. In congenital (infantile) esotropia, the results of symmetrical surgery are excellent. In the older child, less correction can be anticipated from symmetrical surgery than in infancy. After the age of 4, many strabismus surgeons would prefer asymmetric surgery particularly in those cases where the strabismus shows incomitance or strong fixation preference.

Preoperative evaluation

History

This should include details of the pregnancy, birth, milestones, and family history.

Measurement

Measurement is necessary:

- of deviation in primary positions at near and distance and in the other eight positions of gaze

- with and without optical correction

- of maximal deviation under complete dissociation

- of ductions, vergence, forced duction and force generation testing if necessary.

Checklist

It is important first to make certain that:

- the vision is equal

- the pattern of eye movements is constant

- there is no progressive underlying pathology.

Management of specific strabismus syndromes

Amongst the presentations of strabismus in childhood, it is important to realise the associated mechanical restrictions and syndromes.

Duane syndrome

Duane syndrome may be associated with other syndromes and in particular children with Duane's should be assessed for a defect of hearing, skeletal anomalies and features of Goldenhar's syndrome. It is important to realise the exact deficit of movement. Type I may present with the parents expressing concern about a convergent squint because they fail to recognise that the basis of the convergent squint is that one eye is unable to abduct, and the convergent squint is produced by the healthy eye performing a normal adduction movement. In other directions of gaze the child may be binocular; occasionally this is associated with an abnormal head posture which may interfere with school and may require treatment (Figure 7.5). If the child is binocular, surgery should be deferred until school age. Surgery is confined to recession of the medial rectus in one eye and, in severe cases, both eyes. In rare instances, where binocular vision is not present, we have obtained

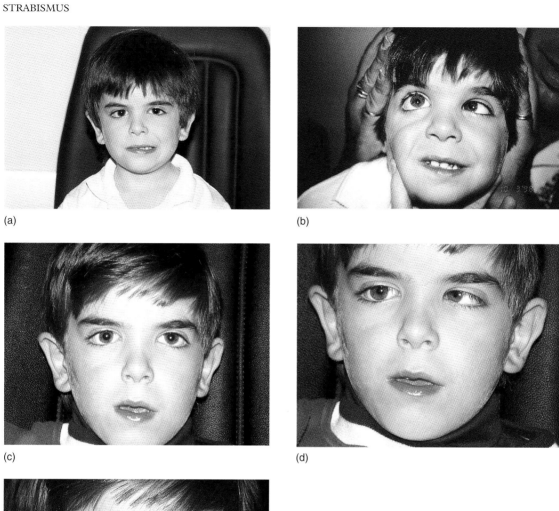

(a)

(b)

(c)

(d)

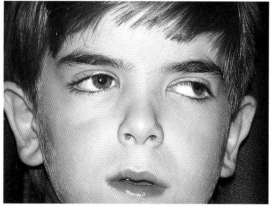

(e)

Figure 7.5 Duane's syndrome Type I in a child who had previous medial and lateral rectus muscle recession with added feature of right facial weakness. Note right convergent squint and face turn to right (a, b). Following the Carlson-Jampolsky procedure (c-e), face turn was abolished and abduction improved. Note limitation of abduction of right eye due to large medial rectus recession (e)

good results from the Carlson–Jampolsky manoeuvre (Figure 7.6). Recession of the antagonist muscle greater than 6 mm will straighten the eye more than 15 dioptres.

Management of "overaction" of the superior oblique or inferior oblique muscle

The basis of this is thought to be a tight lateral rectus muscle slipping over the globe. A posterior fixation along the lateral rectus muscle has been suggested, as has a recession of medial rectus with recession of the lateral rectus of the involved eye. Recession of the lateral rectus in Type I Duane syndrome does not affect the position of the eye in the primary position. Such recession of the lateral rectus seems to also reduce the pseudoptosis sometimes seen in Duane's.

Surgical techniques for Duane syndrome

Most often, the best management of Duane syndrome is not to interfere if there is binocular vision and the patient does not have a marked head posture. Complications of surgery include inducing a cosmetically undesirable exotropia, and still failing to facilitate the patient's ability to abduct the eye. There are children and adults who have enough of a head turn or enophthalmic appearance as to warrant a strabismus repair. In these cases, judicious horizontal muscle surgery may be indicated. In some cases, upshoots and downshoots of the eye occur on adduction. These upshoots and downshoots may be difficult to manage.

Although the aetiology of this problem is debated, most experts would now agree that a tight lateral rectus muscle slips over the globe occasionally when stretched during adduction and slips the eye either up or down, depending on the individual patient.[3,4] When surgery is indicated, a lateral rectus recession or bifurcation of the lateral rectus with superior half transposition up and inferior transposition down may be helpful.[5] It is not due to dysfunction of the superior or inferior oblique muscles.[6] Posterior horizontal fixation procedures will also abolish the upshoots.[7] Amblyopia is rare; however, where Duane's is associated with a marked convergent squint and amblyopia, we have had two cases where an excellent cosmetic result has been obtained with recession of the medial rectus with transposition of the lateral half of the vertical recti and suture beneath the

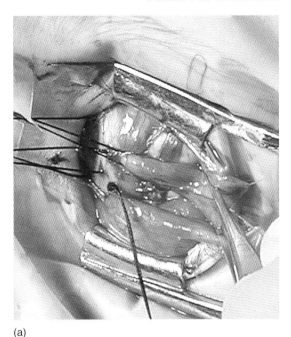

(a)

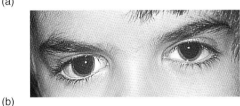

(b)

Figure 7.6 The Carlson–Jampolsky procedure shown involves the separation of the temporal halves of the vertical recti muscles. Joining these two muscle segments, balancing the opposing tone to them and then suturing them together beneath the lateral rectus muscle near its insertion (a) corrected the deviation (as represented in Fig. 7.7). Note the postoperative result (b)

lateral rectus balancing the tone as described in the Carlson–Jampolsky procedure.

Brown syndrome

This is caused by a short, tight superior oblique tendon sheath which prevents the eye from moving upwards in adduction. A forced duction test would distinguish it from an isolated inferior oblique palsy. The majority of patients are straight in primary position and on downgaze for reading.

In attempting to elevate the eyes, they may roll up and out, simulating a V pattern of movement. The parents of the child describe one eye rolling up under the lid. This is the result of Hering's Law. If the eyes are straight in primary gaze and on downgaze, treatment is not advised. Spontaneous resolution has been reported in some cases.

In children with marked head posture and with the affected eye having up to 16 dioptres of hypotropia, tenotomy of the superior oblique tendon and sheath usually improves the vertical deviation, although in some cases overaction of the inferior oblique may occur and require surgery.

The conjunctiva is incised 10 mm from the limbus between medial rectus and superior rectus and the muscle is isolated. Some advise excision of the tendon, preserving the fascial attachments, others advise a silicone expander. Acquired Brown syndrome may be caused by a nodule on the superior oblique tendon preventing smooth passage through the trochlea. The syndrome may also be due to collagen disease, for example rheumatoid arthritis. Such patients often notice a click[8] whilst conservative management with anti-inflammatory agents, including local injection of corticosteroid in the trochlea, is reported to be useful.

Moebius syndrome

Moebius syndrome is diverse in the severity of its presentation. It is thought to result from an ischaemic insult in the first 5–6 weeks of pregnancy. The paresis affects the sixth, seventh, and often bulbar cranial nerves. Moebius syndrome is of interest because it has aplasia of the sixth nerve nucleus in common with Duane syndrome and similarities are reported. The clinical evidence of anomalous innervation of lateral rectus is matched by the frequency of gaze palsies apparent. Although an association is reported, gaze palsies may be overlooked.

Surgery can be surprisingly successful. The possibility of preservation of convergence and substitution of convergent movement on lateral gaze simulating sixth nerve palsy rather than gaze palsy explains some presentations.

Congenital extraocular muscle fibrosis syndrome

This autosomal dominant disorder is also reported as being sporadic. The dominantly inherited group reported by Gillies suggested anomalies in the lateral ventricle.[9] More detailed studies by MRI raise the possibility of a defect in neuronal migration. The bilateral ptosis and complete inability to elevate the eyes limits options for surgery. Although the possibility remains that part of the ptosis is pseudoptosis due to inability to elevate the eyes we have not had much improvement from recession of the inferior recti. In addition to the studies mentioned above, we have seen three sporadic cases. All appear to have normal intelligence. Surgery has not improved them cosmetically.

Strabismus fixus variants of muscle fibrosis syndrome

This condition seen in childhood is characterised by restriction of one or more ocular muscles and may be uniocular. In our experience, the child may fix with the eye with the more restricted movement. This is important to recognise. In one case, a 5-year-old child referred to the university department had marked abnormal head posture with face turn to right, chin down, and marked limitation of movements of the left eye. The eye with restricted movement had not been recognised as the fixing eye and the eye with full movement had been patched, resulting in dense amblyopia. At surgery, a forced duction test to the left eye revealed inability to move the eye from an adducted position and inability to elevate the left eye. Surgery involved tenotomy of left medial rectus, transposition of lateral halves of superior and inferior rectus of the left eye and recession of the medial half of left inferior rectus.

Postoperative abnormal ocular posture was abolished. However, amblyopia of the right eye persisted.

Management of restrictive strabismus in adults

Although thyroid eye disease, myasthenia gravis, and blowout fractures occur in the paediatric age group, they are more common in the older patient.

Myasthenia gravis

Myasthenia gravis is the great mimic and may imitate third nerve palsy with pupil sparing, or internuclear ophthalmoplegia. What is important is to maintain a high index of suspicion for a disease where the treatment is largely in the hands of physicians (see Chapter 5).

Thyroid eye disease

Firstly, treatment principles are that recession is preferred to resection, because resection will further limit restricted movement. Secondly, hangback sutures make surgery in a restricted space more feasible. Finally, adjustable sutures allow more precise adjustment. The common muscles to be limited are the inferior recti and the medial recti. It is important to be mindful of the problems associated with inferior rectus recession.

Treatment of paretic strabismus

Prisms

Prisms may form a useful temporary measure in some cases of thyroid eye disease with muscle involvement, but incomitance is a problem particularly in those cases where the movement may alter depending on the fluctuating involvement of the muscle in thyroid eye disease.

Botulinum toxin

Botulinum toxin may be used in sixth nerve palsies as a temporising manoeuvre. Most would advise waiting up to 6 months to see whether recovery occurs in a nerve palsy. However, if the palsy is complete and appears obvious, for example fracture of the head of the petrous temporal bone, there is a case for considering early surgery.

Surgical principles

If there is not complete palsy, that is in partial weakness of ocular muscles, then weakening the antagonist or the yoke muscle may improve the posture.

In a total ocular muscle palsy, muscle transposition surgery needs to be considered to assist the balancing of the tone of the antagonist. Not doing this results in disappointing outcomes.

Where the ocular tone has changed to produce a concomitant picture, as is seen more frequently in children, consideration may be given to simple recession-resection surgery. Cases seen in adults have their origin in childhood, which may include an acquired sixth nerve palsy which recovers to leave the patient with a concomitant esotropia.

To prevent contracture of the antagonist muscle, intermittent occlusion of the good eye may be helpful, although adults find using the paretic eye a more disorienting experience. If the palsy is not complete, it may be possible for the patient to achieve binocularity with head posture, for example watching television.

Sixth nerve palsy

If there is a complete sixth nerve palsy we have a preference for the Carlson–Jampolsky procedure. This procedure can restore binocular vision. In this instance, having recessed the medial rectus fully on a hangback suture even of 10–12 mm, we perform a conjunctival peritotomy extending from the 12 o'clock to 6 o'clock position to allow access to the outer half of the superior and inferior rectus muscles. A 6-0 vicryl suture is applied to the outer third at its insertion and separated and the lateral halves of the superior and inferior rectus are drawn underneath the lateral rectus (see Figure 7.8). Once joined the tone in the muscles is balanced and the suture inserted. It is important not to allow the muscles to slip behind the equator of the globe and occasionally a suture is used to prevent this.

In incomplete sixth nerve palsy, for example residua of raised intracranial pressure from a sagittal sinus thrombosis, if the child is left with a concomitant esotropia, it can be treated with bilateral medial rectus recession.

Case example A 20-year-old student was involved in a motor vehicle accident with fracture of the base of the skull involving petrous temporal bone, producing a complete sixth nerve palsy. A large medial rectus recession 10 mm with transposition and balance of tone in the lateral half of superior and inferior rectus muscles sutured beneath the lateral rectus restored binocular vision in the primary position. Nine months later the ocular posture was still maintained. The patient was enjoying good binocular vision in the primary position for both near and distance without the need for prism correction, only experiencing diplopia beyond 5° from primary position in the field of the paralysed muscle action.

Third nerve palsy

If a complete third nerve palsy including pupil occurs as a congenital lesion in a child, it is extremely difficult to manage the amblyopia and this may be followed by aberrant regeneration.

The divergent eye can be straightened in a child if the superior oblique with innervation from the trochlear nerve is intact; opposing tone may be created by dislocation of the superior oblique tendon from the trochlea using curved mosquito forceps. The tendon of the superior oblique is then aligned along the upper border of medial rectus, creating a balancing tone to the previously unopposed action of the lateral rectus. This is easier to do in children; in adults, the trochlea may become ossified, so that freeing the tendon is not possible.

Treatment of the ptosis using a silicone sling may be considered. However, exposure keratitis is a real risk because of the absence of a Bell's phenomenon.

If aberrant regeneration is marked, cosmetic improvement is almost impossible.

Fourth nerve palsy

Although superior oblique palsy is common it is important that it be distinguished from skew deviation (frequently associated with other brainstem signs), Brown syndrome, mechanical restriction (blowout fracture or thyroid eye disease) and double elevator palsy (associated pseudoptosis).

Superior oblique muscle paresis is not infrequently bilateral and asymmetrical, particularly after head trauma. This should be suspected if torsion on looking down is more than 10 dioptres. It is important to remember there are two actions to the superior oblique muscle: anterior fibres have a torsional effect and the posterior fibres act as depressors.

Abnormal head posture is usually a manifestation of the torsion, and the Harada-Ito procedure is helpful in treating the excyclotorsion unless complete palsy is present. In marked bilateral superior oblique palsy a bilateral tuck of both superior oblique tendons taking up to 6–8 mm of slack may be performed, recognising the risk of creating a pseudo-Brown syndrome.

In a long-standing fourth nerve palsy there may be contraction in the superior rectus. If on examination there is concomitance, recession of the superior rectus may relieve symptoms. Recognition of torsion can be measured using the double Maddox rod test or the synoptophore.

Treatment of paretic strabismus in children

The third, fourth, and sixth nerve palsies may be encountered in children; they have been reported as congenital lesions. They may be progressive in children and on careful examination, underlying pathology may be found. Congenital third nerve palsy may spare the pupil; where there is pupil paralysis, amblyopia is extremely difficult to avoid, even with intense patching. Testing for a fourth nerve palsy in the presence of a third is important. Excyclotorsion may be suspected with malalignment of the macula relative to the optic disc. Observation of a conjunctival vessel when the child looks down and in may reveal residual torsional action of the superior oblique. The depressor action of the oblique in the presence of a third nerve palsy is frustrated by the divergence.

The fourth nerve is the commonest of the cranial nerves supplying extraocular muscles to be affected and cause disturbance of motility. It may be bilateral and asymmetrical in its presentation. The bilaterality may not be realised until correction of one side. By inducing a vertical deviation, fourth nerve palsy may break down normal binocular vision and if underlying esophoria is present, it may be the underlying cause of the presentation of a convergent squint. In less severe cases, vertical deviations may be compensated for by head posture. Children may develop larger amplitudes of fusion. If there is decompensation in adulthood not controlled by prisms, surgery for weakening the inferior oblique should aim at undercorrection because the patient's fusion capacity can deal with undercorrection but not overcorrection.

Benign sixth nerve palsy of childhood usually occurs in a healthy child following a mild respiratory illness. Its occurrence in an otherwise healthy child and its tendency to resolve justifies the rationale for observation in distinguishing these from brainstem tumours.

Bilateral sixth nerve palsies may represent a false localising sign from causes such as aqueduct stenosis or sagittal sinus thrombosis. It is possible that some cases of congenital esotropia represent transient bilateral sixth nerve palsies although this is difficult to demonstrate or identify as an aetiology.

In considering palsies of the ocular muscles, it is important to remember the differential diagnosis of the congenital absence of a muscle. The recognition of this may occur first at surgery and later be confirmed by MRI or CT scanning.[10]

Specific surgical techniques

The ocular posture of an eye represents a balance of the tone of the extraocular muscles acting upon the globe. The extraocular muscles may be thought of as consisting of antagonistic pairs, and strabismus can be considered to be the result of an imbalance of the antagonistic pairs when the eyes are aligned. From this, the principle of the surgical approach is to restore alignment by weakening one antagonist and/or strengthening the other in its particular direction of action, including changing the direction of muscle action.

Weakening procedures

Recession +/− posterior fixation suture (Faden procedure)

When performing rectus muscle recession (particularly any significant recession) we prefer the hangback suture technique (Figure 7.7). The principle involves the assumption that the muscle is suspended from the insertion together with the assumption that the muscle will gain attachment to the sclera through the insertion without being directly sutured to it. The procedure has the advantage of placing sutures through the thickened insertion stump and the ability to adjust the exact position of the muscle by shortening or lengthening the two sutures suspending each end of the muscle. The further back the recession, the more dangerous the procedure of posterior suture placement especially in myopic eyes or those with thinned sclera. Whilst recession of both medial rectus muscles is often performed for esotropias, the procedure may not only correct any horizontal

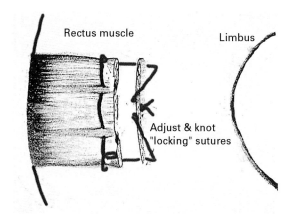

Figure 7.7   Recession with "hang-back" suture

deviation but help in correcting vertical deviation (Figure 7.8).

The value of a posterior fixation suture (Faden procedure) is demonstrated, for example, in those cases where the deviation is greater for near than distance.

Myectomy, marginal myotomy, and tenotomy

The commonest indication for complete myectomy is marked overaction of the inferior oblique muscle. Marginal myotomy is a useful procedure to further weaken a muscle, for example after a bilateral medial rectus recession for congenital esotropia. Complete tenotomy of the superior oblique combined with weakening of the inferior oblique has an accepted place in management of Brown syndrome. Whilst complete myectomy may have a place in marked overaction of the inferior oblique muscle, recession gives more options. In moderate inferior overaction, recession avoids converting inferior oblique overaction with a V pattern to an A pattern. It is also important in the recession of inferior oblique to dissect and isolate the insertion of the muscle (Figure 7.9).

Transposition

Transposition of the horizontal rectus muscles in a vertical direction and changing the

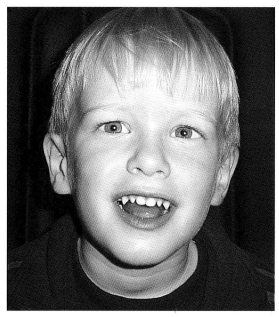

(a)

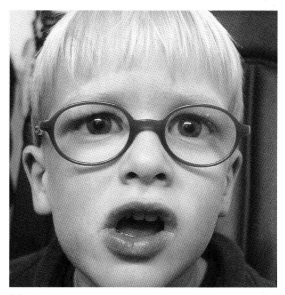

(b)

Figure 7.8   (a) Small residual entropia following initial bilateral medial rectus recession surgery. (b) Fully corrected deviation with glasses postoperatively, in contrast to preoperatively when glasses were of no value.

alignment of horizontal recti is performed in the management of A and V syndromes where there is no obvious oblique dysfunction.

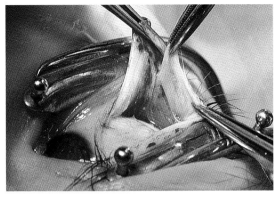

(a)

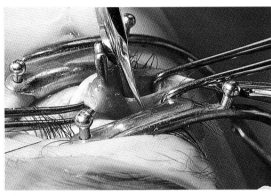

(b)

Figure 7.9   Surgical approach to the inferior oblique insertion. (a) Exposure of the inferior oblique, (b) sharp dissection of the insertion of the inferior oblique muscle prior to recession

Strengthening procedures

Resection +/− advancement

This is the commonest form of strengthening procedure and is commonly performed on the horizontal rectus muscles.

Plication of muscle or its tendon

This procedure is not commonly performed. Plication of the tendon of the superior oblique is most effective in cases of a congenitally lax superior oblique tendon. Caution should be exercised in traumatic fourth nerve palsies because of increased risk of inducing an iatrogenic Brown syndrome.

Transposition

Transposition in a vertical direction of the rectus muscles when overaction of oblique muscles is absent is the commonest method of management of A and V syndromes.

In some cases of isolated complete third nerve palsy, the intact superior oblique muscle with its innervation can be used to provide balancing tone to the lateral rectus, producing improved horizontal alignment.

Vertical muscle surgery in A and V patterns of movements

In congenital esotropia and congenital exotropia, particularly intermittent exotropia, the surgeon's decisions should include whether or not to correct the associated A or V pattern. A and V patterns of movement may be responsible for variability of strabismus.

Scenarios

A and V pattern and evidence of marked overaction of the oblique muscles   The underlying principle is to weaken the overacting muscle. In A exotropia with marked superior oblique overaction, correct with a posterior superior oblique tenotomy leaving the anterior part of the tendon, which controls torsion. Posterior superior oblique tenotomies can collapse the A pattern by as much as 15–20°.

In V exotropia, with marked inferior oblique overaction, correct with inferior oblique muscle weakening procedure.

A and V pattern and no evidence of oblique muscle overaction   The principle is to alter the line of action of the horizontal muscles by vertical shift. Correct by transposition of the horizontal muscles, either moving the medial rectus muscles to the apex of the A or the V or, in the case of lateral rectus muscles,

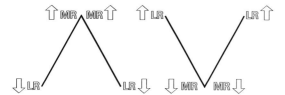

Figure 7.10 Directions to move horizontal recti muscles in A and V patterns of movement: medial recti (MR) towards apex, lateral recti (LR) towards base

moving them towards the base of the A or V (Figure 7.10).

V congenital (infantile) esotropia, with primary inferior oblique overaction and underaction of the superior oblique Correct by weakening the inferior oblique, using myectomy if the inferior oblique overaction is marked. Myectomy may reverse the pattern from a V to an A if inferior oblique overaction is not marked. However, recession of the inferior oblique can be used for marked overaction and it allows a graded operation. If one inferior oblique is overacting more than the other, recession of the inferior obliques can match. Inferior oblique surgery can collapse the V pattern by as much as 15–20°.

V congenital esotropia without overacting obliques Correct with inferior transposition of both medial recti or superior transposition of both lateral recti. These transpositions do not alter the horizontal angles which will need to be addressed separately. They can collapse the pattern by as much as 10–15°.

A pattern movement Superior oblique overaction associated with A pattern movement can be managed with a superior oblique weakening procedure. The procedure preferred is a posterior tenotomy of the superior oblique. Where there is no superior oblique muscle overaction, transposing the rectus muscles

upward or the lateral rectus muscles downward may collapse the pattern by 10–15°.

Management of dissociated vertical deviation (DVD)

The circumstances whereby DVD develops are unknown. It may be exaggeration of the righting reflex seen in lower animals.[19] DVD is characterised by an upward and outward rotation of the eye. Rarely DVD may be present as an addition to oblique dysfunction which will be indicated by the presence of an A or V pattern. DVD must be distinguished from inferior oblique overaction (IOOA). IOOA causes a V pattern and if no V pattern is seen, the diagnosis is purely DVD. Excyclotorsion is an important aspect of DVD and not seen in pure IOOA. Occasional cases of congenital (infantile) esotropia are seen with the combined presence of inferior oblique overaction together with DVD. Helveston drew attention to A pattern exotropia occurring also in combination with DVD. In the above cases, it is wiser to treat horizontal deviation first. With alignment the two elements in the vertical deviation can be treated separately.

The options for management of DVD include the following.

- Recession of the superior rectus preferably on a hangback suture. If fixation in one eye is preferred, unilateral fixation may be performed. The hangback suture may be combined with resection of the inferior rectus.

- The Faden operation on the superior rectus combined with recession of the superior rectus. The presence of the superior oblique muscle adds difficulty to the procedure. The author prefers to place a loop over the muscle rather than suturing it permanently.

- Recession of the inferior oblique muscle with anteriorisation of its insertion. Aligning its insertion temporal to the lateral border of inferior rectus insertion is useful when both DVD and IOOA are present at the same time.[11]

Weakening of the superior oblique

Many cases of A pattern with superior oblique overaction will be improved by a tenotomy of the posterior fibres of the superior oblique. This has the advantage of preserving the anterior torsional fibres of the superior oblique.

Bilateral weakening of superior oblique will cause an esotropic shift of 30–40 D in downgaze for an A pattern, but little horizontal shift in the primary position. If a horizontal deviation is present, it should be addressed in its own right.

Weakening of the inferior oblique

Complete tenotomy may be carried out as part of treatment of a Brown syndrome case. The closer to the trochlea the tendon is severed, the more marked is the response. The procedure may be followed by marked inferior oblique overaction. In cases of overaction of the inferior oblique, we prefer inferior oblique recession as it allows a graded operation.[12] Good results have been reported from lengthening the superior oblique tendon using a silicon "spacer" sutured to the cut ends of the tendon within the sheath.

Secondary overaction of the inferior oblique muscle occurs in patients with superior oblique muscle paresis. The amount of vertical correction is roughly proportional to the degree of preoperative overaction. Weakening of each oblique has little effect on horizontal alignment in the primary position of gaze.[13]

Transposition procedures

Hypotropia A vertical deviation may be treated by a recession–resection procedure of the appropriate vertical rectus muscles.

Double elevator palsy Vertical transposition of both lateral and medial rectus muscles is a useful manoeuvre.

Treatment of superior oblique underaction

Superior oblique underaction is associated with a V pattern of movement. It is important to recognise that in so-called superior oblique palsy, the commonest cause is probably developmental anomalies of the superior oblique and its tendon, and that in paediatric practice the strabismus surgeon will encounter this fairly frequently. Facial asymmetry and photos from childhood will help to identify this group where superior oblique tendon laxity is common. Fourth nerve palsy has been stated to be the commonest isolated nerve palsy faced by the ophthalmologist. In childhood, it must be distinguished from developmental anomaly of the superior oblique. In the neurogenic form, laxity of the tendon is not a feature and there will usually be an event or injury to explain this group. The importance of distinguishing the two groups lies in the different options that the features of these two groups provide for surgical management.

The clinician should consider the torsional and vertical components of superior oblique muscle action. Cases of pure excyclotorsion without hypertropia are best treated with the Harada–Ito procedure. This involves the splitting and anterior transposition of the lateral half of the superior oblique tendon.[14] Acquired large hypertropia may be treated with ipsilateral superior rectus weakening, matching the defect with contralateral inferior rectus weakening. It needs to be appreciated that hypertropias may be treated with inferior oblique recession alone.[15]

Surgical options Underaction of the superior oblique is frequently caused by a maldevelopment of the superior oblique tendon and in some cases absence of the tendon, particularly in those associated with craniofacial dysostoses (Figure 7.11). In this group, undue laxity of the oblique tendon is common and can be demonstrated by exploring the tendon and performing a traction test. It is this group where a tendon tuck is useful and unlikely to induce iatrogenic Brown's syndrome. In superior oblique palsy, weakening of the inferior oblique muscle is the commonest first procedure, being performed in over 90% of cases.[16] For weakening of the contralateral yoke muscle, the inferior rectus is

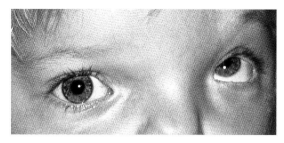

(a)

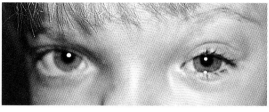

(b)

Figure 7.11 Underaction of left superior oblique in child with left coronal synostosis. Tightening superior oblique tendon laxity improved field of binocular single vision with improved ocular posture without an acquired Brown's syndrome. (a) Preoperative. (b) postoperative

preferred to superior oblique tucks. In neurogenic cases ipsilateral superior rectus recession is useful where a long-standing superior oblique palsy has resulted in tightness of the tendon of the superior rectus. The superior oblique tightening procedure (Harada–Ito) is our preferred option where torsion is the main problem.

Summary of management of A and V patterns

1. Observe the vertical movements of the eyes with accommodation controlled, preferably doing the test at distance and asking the patient to maintain fixation by depressing and elevating the chin. The eyes will move in the opposite directions and measurements can be made.

2. Consider whether the pattern is severe enough to treat.

3. Operate on the superior obliques if overacting in an A pattern and inferior obliques if overacting in a V pattern. If there is no oblique overaction, transpose the horizontal recti, the medial recti to the apex of the pattern, and the lateral recti to the base.

4. Oblique surgery in the adult is less forgiving than in the child.

Adjustable sutures

Adjustable sutures increase the chance of ideal surgical alignment with one operation, decreasing the need for reoperation or staged repairs. More sophisticated surgical techniques and materials have stimulated their increased use. Different techniques involve two-stage procedures where the final alignment is achieved postoperatively with external sutures, or the procedure completed with the patient awake.[17] In our experience, using adjustable sutures has led to better judgement in the operating room, leading to a minority of patients needing further postoperative adjustment (Figure 7.12).

Botulinum chemodenervation

Studies have shown botulinum toxin to be helpful in small to moderate esotropia and exotropia (less than 40 D), active thyroid disease if surgery is inappropriate and postoperative residual strabismus after several weeks. There has been less evidence for use in A and V patterns, DVD or oblique muscle disorders. Success has ranged from 30% to 70% depending on the size of deviation.[18]

Sequelae and complications of strabismus surgery

Anaesthesia

In early childhood, an anaesthetist well experienced in paediatric anaesthesia is essential. Usually day surgery is all that is required. Children need to be prepared for hospital, to have their favourite toy with them and to have their parents with them during induction and there for them when they awake. Surgeons need to constantly be aware of the oculocardiac reflex, particularly early in the operation.

For patients known to be at risk of malignant hyperthermia who require a general anaesthetic, agents such as halothane and succinyl choline muscle relaxants should be avoided. Malignant hyperthermia is a rare hereditary disorder characterised by gross hypermetabolic state in skeletal muscle and may be fatal. Unexpected tachycardia and pyrexia under anaesthesia may indicate malignant hyperthermia.

Ocular alignment

Ocular alignment may be anticipated in 85% of straightforward cases. Failure to respond as anticipated reflects the reality that biological responses are not 100% predictable. Informed consent of the patient and parents should include explanation that departures from the anticipated response are not complications but part of the natural history of the condition, which in most cases are readily dealt with by a further procedure. It is important for the clinician to be aware of the risk of inducing an A pattern by confusion of DVD with inferior oblique overaction and weakening of the inferior oblique muscle. Other risks include operating without taking account of the patient's accommodation in accommodative squint or intermittent exotropia. Alignment problems may cause postoperative diplopia, including thyroid patients who still have active disease.

Overcorrection of exo or eso deviations is perhaps the commonest alignment problem to consider. The younger the child, the more at risk is any potential for binocular vision with fusion. The more mature the visual system, the greater the risk of persistent diplopia. Clinical decisions can be difficult. For example, a child of 2 years presents with intermittent exotropia. Such cases often have excellent fusion potential with normal binocular vision and bifoveal fusion for near. Early surgery may result in overcorrection,

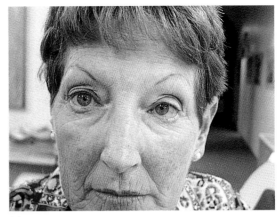

(a)

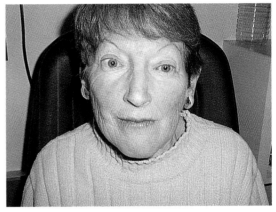

(b)

Figure 7.12 This patient had a long-standing left sixth nerve palsy associated with hypertension, development of cataract and reduced vision from 6/12 to 6/60. She had a 15° strabismus corrected by medial rectus recession using adjustable sutures with a good cosmetic result

esotropia, disruption of fusion and amblyopia. If it is a small overcorrection the result may be microsquint with retention of peripheral fusion, monofixation syndrome and loss of bifoveal fusion for near although more constant alignment at distance. On the other hand deferring surgery until after age 4 years is more likely to be associated with retention of bifoveal fusion for near but less stable deviation for distance. In the older patient with a mature visual system overcorrection will be accompanied by more persistent diplopia. It is in this group of patients that the argument for adjustable sutures is strongest. The alignment can be corrected in the ward or the clinic under local anaesthesia.

Lost or slipped muscles

The fascial connections between the oblique muscles and the inferior, lateral and superior rectus muscles make recovery of any one of these muscles easier than the medial rectus, which is the commonest muscle to lose its attachments completely. In our experience in nearly every case, a lost medial rectus muscle remains in the sub-Tenon's space, and a careful search with the operating microscope should be made, though the muscle may be found as far back as the optic nerve. The surgeon should be extremely cautious venturing outside Tenon's capsule and disturbing the orbital fat and particularly allowing fat into the sub-Tenon's space which may result in adhesion syndromes.

If sutures are not tied tightly, marked limitation of abduction may be present on the first postoperative day. It is important to return to surgery promptly following diagnosis, as contraction and fibrosis may occur; however, in our experience, patients present with lost muscles even 20 years later.

Case example

A 28-year-old nurse presented as an adult with a history of sudden onset of divergent squint following surgery for convergent squint as a child. The patient was still distressed at the appearance and limited ability to adduct the eye. The patient had had unsuccessful exploration to retrieve the lost medial rectus followed by eight subsequent surgeries on other ocular muscles with an outcome she still regarded as cosmetically unsatisfactory. With the advantage of the operating microscope and good illumination, exploration of the sub-Tenon's space revealed the medial rectus muscle on the medial side of the left eye 2 mm from the optic nerve. Although some gliosis and contracture

had occurred, it was still possible with the microscope to recover the muscle and reattach it 10 mm from the limbus with a dramatic improvement in ocular posture, although there was an incomitance because of residual contracture in the muscle.

Slipped muscles within the muscle sheath

Slippage of muscles within the muscle sheath is difficult to recognise initially, as in the immediate postoperative period the eyes may look reasonably straight or slightly divergent. A month or two later, for example in the case of medial rectus recession, the divergence is worse, and the muscle is underacting even more. Risk of inferior rectus muscle slippage needs emphasis because it may go unrecognised. Reoperation may be misleading as careful surgery may reveal the sheath of the muscle appropriately attached to the sclera, and the surgeon may be misled into thinking that he or she is dealing with an attenuated muscle. It is important to continue to explore the muscle and the bunched up muscle further back in the sheath must be grasped and reattached. Again some incomitance of movement may be the result of contracture if surgery is done late.

Restriction of upgaze after inferior oblique muscle weakening surgery

This has been referred to as an adherence syndrome.[15] The usual explanation is breaching Tenon's capsule with the disturbance of fat and bleeding. Surgery is almost always required and inferior rectus recession is effective. The forced duction test may be positive. The complication is avoided with careful separation of the inferior oblique from Tenon's capsule and being careful to keep the muscle hook from tearing the capsule.

Hazards of inferior rectus recession

The objective of recession of the inferior oblique muscle must include the patient's ability to maintain fusion in downgaze. This may mean the patient is left with slight chin up in the primary position. Fusion in downgaze is important in reading and going down stairs. In a restrictive problem like thyroid eye disease which makes the patient orthophoric in primary position, correcting the hypotropia by weakening the inferior rectus is associated with a different set of problems, including diplopia in downgaze. In several cases, we have resorted to combining weakening the muscle without further altering its insertions by marginal myotomy. This has been done as a secondary procedure if the initial surgery was unsuccessful.

Hazards of inferior rectus recession include recession of the lower lid. Caution must be exercised if the inferior rectus is recessed by more than 3 mm. If the inferior rectus is recessed more than 3 mm, even with careful dissection of the check ligaments, lower lid retraction will follow. At review 1–2 months later, surgery may be indicated using eyebank sclera grafted to the lower end of the tarsal plate to reposition the lid and raise the level of the lower lid.

It is important to operate when the patient is euthyroid and the thyroid eye disease is quiescent. Even so, recession of the inferior rectus may be followed by conversion of the hypotropia to hypertropia if there is involvement of the superior rectus. Subsequent forced duction testing will show that the superior rectus is also involved and this can be further confirmed with imaging.

Globe perforation

The surgeon should be alert to this possibility, especially in the thinned area of sclera immediately posterior to the insertion of the muscle. The increasing popularity of hangback sutures for medial and lateral rectus muscle surgery should reduce the risk of perforation. If perforation occurs with loss of vitreous, a small area of cryotherapy should be performed visualising the area through a dilated pupil, and subconjunctival antibiotics at the conclusion of

the surgery may be equally wise. The risk of retinal detachment is small; however, a retinal surgeon should be consulted. The risk of perforation includes endophthalmitis.

Postoperative infection

Endophthalmitis

Endophthalmitis is rare, but may occur. A retinal surgeon should be consulted, with a vitreous biopsy and instillation of intravitreal antibiotics instituted as a matter of urgency.

Orbital cellulitis

Undue swelling of the upper and lower lid with fever and pain on eye movement requires urgent admission. Smear and blood cultures should be performed and systemic intravenous antibiotic should be administered.

Conjunctivitis

Topical antibiotics should be used for 1–2 weeks. Prophylaxis by instillation of half strength povidone-iodine may also help prevent perioperative conjunctivitis.[16,17]

Tenon's capsule inflammation

Prolapse of Tenon's capsule into the conjunctival wound can be associated with inflammation. Careful closure of conjunctiva and the use of saline will distinguish Tenon's from conjunctiva.

Suture granuloma and suture abscess

These may present as a tender lump and if not resolving, should be excised preferably after 10 days of surgery. Replacement of suture is rarely required. Allergic reactions to polyglycolic acid sutures are rare, and more common with catgut. Skin tests by threading the suture through the skin will confirm this.

Epithelial conjunctival inclusion cysts

These are rare, but may reach a large size and should be removed under the operating microscope. Inflammation of the conjunctiva can occur if Tenon's layer is breached and fat prolapses forward. Prophylaxis is preferred.

Redundant conjunctiva

Redundant conjunctiva may require excision. Care when suturing the conjunctiva to the limbus is important. If it disturbs the tear film, discomfort and thinning of the cornea (dellen) may occur.

Conjunctival scarring and displacement of plica

This usually occurs after multiple procedures. It is probably best dealt with by excision of the plica and a simple conjunctival graft beneath the upper anterior to the superior rectus.

Anterior segment ischaemia syndrome

Patients may present within 24 hours of surgery with corneal oedema and a mild anterior uveitis and may respond to topical or systemic corticosteroids. The anterior ciliary vessels supplying anterior segment structures run superficial within the four recti muscle sheaths. Removal of recti may predispose the anterior segment to ischaemia, especially in older patients over the age of 60 with a past history of systemic vascular disease. Surgery involving three or more recti at the same time or within 6 months has a higher risk of ischaemia. It is also possible to perform surgery preserving the anterior ciliary vessels.[18] Anterior ischaemia is uncommon in children.

References

1. Kutschke PJ. Use of prisms: are they really helpful? *Am Orthoptics J* 1996;**46**:61–4.
2. Sinelli JM, Repka MX. Prism treatment of incomitant horizontal deviations. *Am Orthoptics J* 1996;**41**:123–6.
3. Cassidy L, Taylor D, Harris C. Abnormal supranuclear eye movements in the child: a practical guide to examination and interpretation. *Surv Ophthalmol* 2000;**44**:479–506.
4. Kraft SP. A surgical approach for Duane's syndrome. *J Paediatr Ophthalmol Strabismus* 1988;**25**:119–30.
5. Carlson MR, Jampolsky A. An adjustable transposition procedure for abduction deficiencies. *Am J Ophthalmol* 1979;**87**:382–7.
6. Magoon E, Cruciger M, Scott AB. Diagnostic injection of xylocaine into extra-ocular muscles. *Ophthalmology* 1982;**89**:489–91.
7. von Noorden GK, Murray E. Up and downshoot in Duane's retraction syndrome. *J Paediatr Ophthalmol Strabismus* 1986;**23**:212–15.
8. Knapp P. A and V patterns. In: Burian HM, ed. *Symposium on Strabismus*. St Louis: Mosby, 1971.
9. Fierson WM, Boger WP, Diorio PC. The effect of bilateral superior oblique tenotomy on horizontal deviation in A-pattern strabismus. *J Paediatr Ophthalmol Strabismus* 1980;**17**:364–71.
10. Stager DR, Parks MM. Inferior oblique weakening procedures. Effect on primary position horizontal alignment. *Arch Ophthalmol* 1973;**90**:15–16.
11. Harada M, Ito Y. Surgical correction of cyclotropia. *Jpn J Ophthalmol* 1964:88–96.
12. Helveston EM. Surgery of the superior oblique muscle. In: Helveston EM, ed. *Symposium on Strabismus*. St Louis: Mosby, 1978.
13. Wright KW. Adjustable suture technique. In: Wright KW, ed. *Colour Atlas of Ophthalmic Surgery*. Philadelphia: Lippincott, 1992.
14. Biglan AW, Burnstine RA, Rogers GL. Management of strabismus with botulinum A toxin. *Ophthalmology* 1989;**96**:935–43.
15. Parks MM. The weakening surgical procedures for eliminating overaction of the inferior oblique muscle. *Am J Ophthalmol* 1972;**73**:107–22.
16. Apt L, Isenberg S, Yoshimori R, Spierer A. Outpatient topical use of povidone-iodine in preparing the eye for surgery. *Ophthalmology* 1989;**96**:289.
17. Apt L, Isenberg S, Yoshimori R, Paez JH. Chemical perforation of the eye in ophthalmic surgery: effect of povidone-iodine on the eye. *Arch Ophthalmol* 1984;**102**:728.
18. McKeown CA, Lambert M, Shore JW. Preservation of anterior ciliary vessels during extraocular muscle surgery. *Ophthalmology* 1989;**96**:498.
19. Brodsky MC. Dissociated vertical divergence: a righting reflex gone wrong. *Arch Ophthalmol* 1999;**117**:1216–22.

Glossary

AC:A ratio The ratio of accommodation produced by convergence to the accommodation measured in prism dioptres.

Amblyopia An acquired defect in monocular vision due to disturbed binocular vision without an underlying organic cause.

Angle kappa The angle between the line joining the visual axis (the line between the fovea and object of interest) and the mid-pupillary line.

Anomalous retinal correspondence Where the fovea of one eye is paired with a non-foveal part of the fellow deviated eye to acquire a common visual direction.

Binocular single vision Using two eyes simultaneously with bifoveal fixation to form a common single precept.

Consecutive strabismus Refers to reversal of direction of strabismus usually as a result of surgery.

Diplopia and confusion *Diplopia* is the simultaneous perception of two images of a single object. *Confusion* is the simultaneous appreciation of two superimposed images that cannot be fused into a single precept.

Fusion Involves a sensory and a motor component. There is integration of the two dissimilar images from each eye into a single precept, which is maintained through motor responses involving the ocular muscles.

Head thrusting A feature of clinical motor apraxia. The child unable to initiate saccade maintains fixation on initial object of regard. To break fixation the head is turned and the eyes are dragged from object of regard to fresh object of regard. To centre the gaze the head is turned back in the opposite direction, completing the appearance of head thrusting.

Monofixation syndrome A sensory monocular status where there is an absence of bifoveal central binocular fusion in the presence of peripheral binocular fusion. The absence of central fusion is associated with a central scotoma in one eye during the act of binocular viewing.

Near reflex A reflex where there is pupil constriction and convergence linked to accommodation.

Optokinetic mechanism Where the image of the object of regard is held steady on the retina during sustained head rotation.

Primary position of gaze The position of both eyes looking straight ahead with the body and head erect.

Saccade A refixation movement, bringing the object of regard onto the fovea.

Smooth pursuit Holding the image of a moving object on the fovea.

Stereopsis The binocular perception of depth.

Strabismus Malalignment of the eyes owing to a breakdown or failure of development of binocular single vision at a particular test distance or in a particular direction of gaze. *Incomitant strabismus* is where the angle of misalignment of a strabismus, measured at a particular test distance, varies depending on the direction of gaze. *Concomitant strabismus* is where with the accommodation controlled, the angle of misalignment of the strabismus when examined at a particular test distance will remain constant regardless of the direction of gaze.

Vergence movement A disjunctive movement. Both eyes move in opposite directions to keep object of regard focused on each fovea simultaneously.

Vestibular mechanism Where the image of the object of regard is held on the retina during brief head rotation.

Visual fixation With the head stationary, visual fixation is the act of focusing a stationary object of regard upon the fovea.

Index

Page numbers in **bold** refer to figures and those in *italic* type refer to tables or boxed material. Abbreviations used as sub entries include; DVD dissociated vertical deviation, MFS, monofixation syndrome and OKN, optokinetic nystagmus.

abscesses 89
AC:A ratios, accommodative esotropia 28, 30
accommodation 3
accommodative esotropia 4, 28
  AC:A ratios 28, 30
  acquired in children 28–31
  age of onset 28
  convergence excess 30
  differential diagnosis 30
  fully accommodative 29, **29**
  management 28, 30, 73, **73**
  myopia 29, 30, 73
  partially accommodative **29,** 29–30, **30**
active force generation test 67
adherence syndrome 88
adjustable sutures 86, **87**
adult strabismus 21–2, 47–54
  acquired esotropia 29
  adaptations 48
  aetiological causes 21–2, 48
    convergence insufficiency 53
    muscular 51–2
    neurological 52–3
    restrictive 50–1
    secondary 17
    skew deviation 53
    surgical 51
  childhood origin 47–8
  childhood *versus* 47
  decompensation 17

  examination 48, 49–50, 67–9
  history 48
  incomitant 4
  loss of fusion, significance 17
  neurological examination/imaging 29
  sequelae 15–16
    diplopia *see* diplopia
    suppression 16, **16**
    visual confusion 15, **15,** 49
  sudden onset 17
  see also specific types
albinism, congenital nystagmus 43
alternate cover test 65
alternating divergent strabismus 35, **35**
amblyopia 14, 21, 23–4
  accommodative esotropia 28
  aetiology 14
  concept 5–6, 70
  critical periods 14, 71, 73
  diagnosis 72
  iatrogenic 24, 72
  management
    non-surgical 71–2
    principles 23, 72
  see also individual types
amblyoscope 63
anaesthesia complications 86–7
aniseikonia 23
anisometropic amblyopia 5–6, 14, 23
  critical period 73
anomalous retinal correspondence (ARC) 14–15, **15**
anterior segment ischaemia syndrome 90
AO vectograph 62
A patterns 4–5, **5**
  congenital esotropia 4, 24, 26
  congenital exotropia 83

93

vertical muscle surgery 83–6, **84, 86**
weakening 81–2, **83,** 84
see also individual muscles; specific procedures
timing of 17
sutures
adjustable 86, **87**
complications 89
"hang back" 51, 81, **82**
synoptophore 63

Teller tests 8, **8,** 61
tenon's capsule 88, 89
tenotomy 82, 84
Tensilon test *52*
third cranial nerve 9
aberrant regeneration 38, **38,** 52, 80
divisions 52
muscles innervated 10
palsies 38, **38,** 52–3
congenital 81
management 80, 81
thyroid eye disease 50–1
management 51, 79
Titmus Fly test 62
toys, visual acuity testing 60, **60**
transient skew deviation 41
transposition procedures 82, 83, 84, 85
trochlear injury 51
tropia 65

vascular disease, degenerative 22
vergence 11
definition 13
examination 69
functions *12*
vestibulo–ocular reflex 11, 13
assessment 61, 69
definition 13
function *12*
vision
colour 61
defects 58
development *see* visual development

double *see* diplopia
near reflex 3–4
normal binocular *see* binocular vision
sensory pathways 7–8, **8**
visual acuity testing 68
babies/young infants 8, **8,** 60–1
cycloplegic refraction 61, **61**
fixation 60, **60**
small objects **60,** 60–1
stereoacuity 33, 62
toys used for testing 60, **60**
see also specific methods
visual confusion 15, **15,** 49
visual cortex
extrastriate 8–9
ocular dominance columns 18
striate (primary V1) 8
visual development 3, 17
critical periods 5, 6, 9, 14, 17
deprivation effects 6, 8–9, 14, 18
amblyopia *see* amblyopia
M and P pathways 9
plasticity 6, 14
sensory–motor integration 7, **7,** 8–9
timescale 14
visual field, suppression of *see* suppression
visual (sensory) processing 7–8, **8**
cortical 8
integration 8–9
LGN 8
magnocellular (M) stream 7, **8,** 9, 17
parvocellular (P) stream 7, **8,** 9
retina 7–8
V patterns 4–5, **5**
Brown's syndrome **40,** 78
congenital esotropia 4, 24, 25, 26, 84
congenital exotropia 32, 83
fourth nerve palsy 53, 85
surgical correction 83–6
see also A patterns

Worth 4-dot test
fusion assessment 62, **63**